Sick of Being Sick

Sick
of Being
Sick

*The Woman's Holistic
Guide to Conquering
Chronic Illness*

Brenda Walding, DPT, FDN-P

NEW YORK

LONDON • NASHVILLE • MELBOURNE • VANCOUVER

Sick of Being Sick

The Woman's Holistic Guide to Conquering Chronic Illness

Published in New York, New York, by Morgan James Publishing in partnership with Difference Press. Morgan James is a trademark of Morgan James, LLC.
www.MorganJamesPublishing.com

ISBN 9781642794656 paperback
ISBN 9781642794663 eBook
Library of Congress Control Number: 2019933107

Cover & Interior Design by:
Christopher Kirk
www.GFSstudio.com

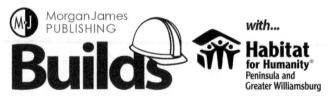

Morgan James is a proud partner of Habitat for Humanity Peninsula and Greater Williamsburg. Partners in building since 2006.

Get involved today! Visit
MorganJamesPublishing.com/giving-back

*To all the beautiful women of the world
who have ever struggled and suffered
as a result of chronic illness.
May this book lead you back to your heart
and remind you of the power you
hold within you to heal.*

Table of Contents

Note: Dear reader, please note that I've used the word "God" and several others descriptive synonyms for God in this book. If you get hung up on the word "God" or any of the others I use, please substitute the name that feels good to you and symbolizes your Higher Power. Other names I've used in this text: Source, Infinite Power, Creative Consciousness, Divine Intelligence, the Divine, Spirit, the Infinite, and Love. Namaste!

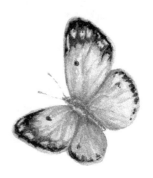

Foreword

I first met Brenda a few years ago when she came to me for guidance and a strong desire to take a natural and holistic approach to dealing with her breast cancer diagnosis. It has been an honor to support her on her healing path and I'm so inspired by how much she has grown, healed and transformed during this time. As she describes in her book, she truly has used this "disease as a divine opportunity" to dive deep into her heart, reclaim her power and health and create a life of even deeper meaning, connection, joy and purpose. And you can too! I know this because I've experienced this first-hand in my life and have witnessed and supported hundreds of women who have healed from cancer and chronic illness. In fact, my own breast cancer diagnosis was the catalyst that led me down an extraordinary path of self-discovery, healing, and transformation and ultimately awakened me to my passion to empower other women to heal naturally from breast cancer.

In a day and age when chronic illness is present in such epidemic proportions, we need to stop and take a deeper look at what's going on and implement strategies that get to the root of the matter. That's why this is such an important book, because it provides a comprehensive, holistic and heart-centered approach to overcoming chronic illness. No matter what chronic health issue or illness you are facing, the 9 Whole-Hearted Healing Essentials in this book will guide you on your unique path, empower you to take control of your own healing, lead you back to your heart and remind you of the power you hold within you to heal. This book contains practical tools, concepts and crucial information required to not only heal, but to create a life you love and deserve. It moves beyond nutrition and lifestyle advice and dives into key topics that are often overlooked or missing, but essential, for any woman desiring to truly heal.

I love and appreciate how Dr. Walding shares her decade-long healing journey and recovery from a place of such genuine authenticity and openness. All of us who have experienced the struggles, challenges, fear, overwhelm, and devastation that often accompanies chronic health issues can relate to her story. Her triumph over such adversity provides a beacon of hope and practical tools for all women that feel lost, afraid and alone.

As a holistic breast cancer doctor, I have come to know and understand through my own research and healing journey, the absolute importance of learning to access the power of the heart to heal. I love how Brenda's Whole-Hearted Healing approach focuses on learning to navigate our health and lives by tapping into the wisdom of the heart, which is something we must learn to do in order to heal and thrive on the individual and collective level.

Sick of Being Sick, is truly a love letter, a roadmap and a gift to ALL women desiring to reclaim their health and live their best life possible. As you navigate the pages of this book, do so with an open mind and heart and let Dr. Walding's words be your guidance and assurance that illness can be the catalyst to experiencing greater health, happiness and harmony in your life!

Dr. Véronique Desaulniers, DC

Founder of Breast Cancer Conqueror® and The 7 Essentials System®

Author of Amazon #1 Best Seller, *Heal Breast Cancer Naturally*

Introduction

"The natural healing force within each of us
is the greatest force in getting well."
– Hippocrates

W*hy is this happening to me?*
When is this nightmare going to end?
What's it going to take for me to be well again?

If you're like me, you've asked yourself these question thousands of times and despite your focused efforts, you've failed to find the answers. You wake every morning and realize you still have the same debilitating symptoms, maybe it's pain, fatigue, anxiety, or (fill in the blank). For some, you've been given a dreaded diagnosis that lurks in every corner of your mind and weighs heavy on your heart.

You've been to conventional medical doctors, taken the pills, tried the treatments, and still don't feel much better – and possibly feel even worse. You've begun to explore other options. You've dabbled in different diets, tried the "magic potions," swallowed fistfuls of supplements, bought a juicer, and maybe even started doing yoga. You may have gotten some results, but you still don't feel *well*. Have you googled "how to heal yourself" in a desperate attempt for answers, only to wind up more confused and utterly overwhelmed by the sheer volume of often contradictory information that makes you want to smack your head up against the wall? It feels nearly impossible to know who to trust, what to do, and who to listen to.

Living with chronic health issues may feel like a never-ending nightmare with no real promise of resolution. For years I remember feeling like I was drowning, desperate for a life preserver to pull me safely to shore where I could bask in the sun and take a full breath without feeling like my lungs were going to collapse. Chronic illness can be pervasive and all-consuming. It often impacts *every* single aspect of a women's life, *every* single day, and for some, *every* single hour, minute, and second.

For many it's the physical symptoms – the pain or fatigue or perhaps rashes, hair loss, low libido, insomnia, digestive upset, headaches (or a combination of many ailments) that suck the enjoyment out of just about everything and keep you from being able to do the things you love to do. You may struggle with how the symptoms affect your physical appearance – feeling a sense of self-loathing, unworthiness, and lack of confidence every time you look in the mirror or see yourself in photographs. Your friends don't get it, your family doesn't get it, and it feels like no one gets what it's like to be you. It's hard to relate to others because not only do they not get it, you don't want to burden them, you don't want them to feel sorry for you, and you don't want to pretend to be bright and shiny and happy when you're not. And although you crave intimacy and connection, you isolate yourself and feel very, very alone.

I remember a rare occasion when I ventured out to a dinner gathering with some friends while I was in the thick of the intensive cancer treatments I was receiving. I was surrounded by people, but I had never felt so alone. Moms complained about how their children wouldn't go down for naps after too much sugar at Disney Land the day before or how their yearly Costco membership went up by twenty dollars. "Seriously?!" I thought. I couldn't relate one iota. Tears stung the corners of my eyes and I wanted to scream. I would've given *anything* for these to be my biggest complaints. I stood there with a tumor growing in my breast, feeling such anguish and grief, and wondering if I would ever be able to have kids. I said nothing, forced a smile, and politely excused myself to get some air. Sometimes when you are sick, lonely follows you no matter where you go and no matter who are you with.

Illness often impacts a woman's professional life, as well as her relationships. Can you relate? Some women have to quit their jobs or scale back. Others push through but struggle to keep up like they used to. Pain, lack of mental clarity, or brain fog can have real effects on your ability to perform at work. The strain that disease can have on a marriage, partnership, and family can be devastating. I know several women with cancer whose partners left them due to the unbearable strain it was on their relationship. I'm grateful my marriage weathered the storms, but, man, was it challenging. Many women struggle to nurture their partner and care for their children the way they want to, while still trying to care for and heal themselves. It's a constant juggling act that almost always ends up with you collapsing on the floor in a hot mess of dropped balls, self-criticism, and frustrated tears.

Now ... let's talk about the fear. It's the fear, doubt, and overwhelm that keep you stuck and make it hard to fully participate in life. The barrage of questions in your mind is a cacophony that keeps you from finding the peace and clarity you so desperately desire. Am I going to have to live like this forever? What's wrong with me? Am I being punished? Am I going to die? How do I make this go away? Which doctor should I use? Should I try that program? Should I take that supplement? Does my partner think I'm ugly? Will I ever be happy again? And it just keeps going like machine gun rapid-fire. It can literally paralyze you and keep you feeling sorry for yourself for days and months on end. Especially if you have been given a scary diagnosis and/or dismal prognosis, fear can hang over you like a black cloud, making it hard to make decisions or find much peace or joy in your life. You know that staying here will not get you well, but you aren't sure how to shake it.

And if all this wasn't enough, medical bills, alternative and holistic therapies and treatments, diets, supplements, and medications can drain your bank account, creating additional stress on you, your family, and your entire life. I know what it's like to lose your home and entire savings in order pay for a treatment that you hope will save your life. Dealing with chronic illness can feel like a black hole that not only sucks away your finances, but your dreams and happiness too.

You know that staying stuck in this never-ending nightmare could cost you everything – your life, your sanity, your happiness, your dreams, your fulfillment, and possibly your relationship, family, job, and financial freedom. Maybe it already has. But, it doesn't have to be that way. And although sometimes you feel like giving up and resigning to the fact that being sick and miserable is just the way it's gonna be, you have a flicker of hope – a light – that reminds you that you were meant to be well, to thrive, and to live your dreams. Hang on to that light, dear soul – it's your way out of this nightmare.

Can you move beyond the prison of this chronic illness or the persistent health challenges in your life?

Yes, I believe you can. And I believe you can move beyond this disease and create a life that you love, because I've experienced it. I've met, studied, and learned from other people and healers who have experienced it too. The truth is that instead of illness being the greatest stumbling block in your life, it can be an even greater stepping stone to a life of greater richness and meaning.

What if the obstacle is the way?

What if this disease is your divine opportunity to transform your life, to live better than you ever have, and to love deeper than you knew was possible?

What if this disease was your sacred springboard, launching you into an experience of greater joy, peace, connection, freedom, and fulfillment that your soul has always craved, but you have yet to experience?

It took me a decade of suffering, a run-in with cancer, and a deep dive into my heart to experience this. I've learned that I can move beyond the stranglehold of disease and create a rich and meaningful life. For this awareness, I am grateful. And this is what I know is possible for you too, if you choose it.

This book is my love letter to you … and every woman who has crossed my path and every woman that I have yet to meet who is struggling to heal and be well. This is the book I would've handed myself ten years ago – to the broken, miserable, emaciated woman lying in bed covered in rashes, who could barely get up the stairs. However, I know that everything that has happened leading up to this moment got me to where I am today and I wouldn't change a thing. I honor all the pain, all the struggle, all the learning, all the growth, all the heartache and all the tears that have led me to this moment in time when I am writing these words to you. Because for the first time ever, I can say that I know who I really am, I love myself, I love my life, and I feel a sense of wholeness I had not known, but always craved. Does this mean my life is perfect or that I don't encounter fear or challenges or that I feel amazing all the time? No … but there's a deeper sense of peace, joy, purpose, vitality, connection, and fulfillment I have not known before. And I know that I am here to help you find that too.

Think of this book as a roadmap, with me as your guide – to healing, to wholeness, and to the place in your heart where you know who you really are. In the following pages, I will share my journey, help you uncover blind spots that are sabotaging your healing, and teach you my Whole-Hearted Healing approach. This holistic, heart-centered approach to healing and thriving consists of 9 Essentials that have been "essential" to my healing journey, as well as those of countless other women, and it will assist you in your quest for vibrant health and creating a life that you love.

Whole-Hearted Healing Essentials

Essential #1 – Taking Responsibility for Your Health

Essential #2 – Creating a Vision: Harnessing Your Power to Heal

Essential #3 – Thoughts and Beliefs

Essential #4 – Feel Your Feelings

Essential #5 – Eat, Drink, Detox

Essential #6 – Live to Thrive: Key Lifestyle Habits

Essential #7 – Connection and Relationships

Essential #8 – Love Yourself

Essential #9 – Trust and Surrender

First, you will learn the importance of taking responsibility for your health. Next, you will learn how to create a vision for your health and life and harness the power of your thoughts, words, feelings, and beliefs. This is super powerful! Then we will dive into the importance of feeling your feelings, healing emotional wounds, and cultivating emotional intelligence. I will discuss how to reduce toxin exposure in your environment, which lifestyle habits you'll want to make sure you address, the importance of food as medicine, which foods to avoid, and the importance of digestion, hydration, and detoxification. You will learn the vital importance of loving yourself and properly nourishing and caring for yourself, and learn to live your life from a place of trust and surrender. Then finally, we will discuss where the rubber meets the road – key things to focus on as you begin to implement these 9 Essentials on a daily basis, as well as common obstacles you may face along your path that may hold you back from getting the results you desire.

Before we dive into the Whole-Hearted Healing framework and the 9 Essentials, I want to take some time to share a little about my own personal healing journey.

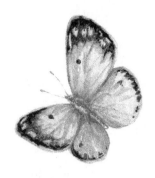

Chapter 1:

My Journey

*"Remember that wherever your heart is,
there you will find your treasure."*
– Paulo Coelho, *The Alchemist*

O ver a decade ago I was lying in my bed in the middle of the
day covered in ice packs. Ice packs on my legs, ice packs on my
arms, and some on my torso. For months and months on end
numbing my skin with ice was the only way I could sleep or get any relief
from the pain and the itching. My body was covered in rashes – oozing,
red, angry rashes. Looking in the mirror at my sunken eyes, bony frame,
and my red splotchy skin made me feel so sad and disgusted that I made a
point to avoid all mirrors in order to keep from breaking down into tears.
It was difficult to eat and hurt to swallow because I had pus-filled lesions
on the inside of my mouth and throat. The infection was making me
weaker and weaker and the medications weren't working. My head ached,
my body throbbed, my hair was falling out, and I had a hard time getting
up and down the stairs to our condo on the second floor. I was home alone
in the middle of the day because I was a woman on medical disability in

her late twenties. *How could this really be happening to me?* I thought. *What on earth did I do to deserve this?* Every single thing I had going for me – everything I had prided myself on being – was stripped away from me. The beautiful, smart, successful athlete and physical therapist was gone. I wasn't exactly sure who I was anymore. All I knew was that I was the "sick girl" who was grieving the loss of the woman she used to be.

Prior to this moment, I never understood why anyone would want to take their own life. I couldn't understand how things could ever get bad enough to end it all – until now. I wouldn't say I was suicidal, but I laid there and gave God a little piece of my mind. If I'm going to have to keep living like this, I'd rather you go ahead and take me now. This is most certainly no way to live. I'm good. I'm ready to go. There is no point in me being here any longer. Oh, and I'm pissed, by the way. This is pretty cruel, isn't it? What did I do to deserve this? I heard nothing in response.

Leading up to my downward health spiral, I considered myself quite healthy and was successful in many areas of my life. I had been a highly-decorated athlete (a basketball and soccer player most of my life) and was an extremely bright student. I had a room full of trophies, awards, and medals. I worked hard to excel at everything – always wanting to please my parents, peers, teachers, and coaches. I often played on several sports teams simultaneously while juggling school and time with my friends. While other kids were going off on summer vacations, I hit the track, weight room, or soccer field to train. To say I was dedicated was an understatement. I look back on that now and realize that the motivation behind most of my efforts was deeply rooted in a desire to "be perfect" and to get approval from others, although I didn't realize it then. I was looking outside of myself for love and worthiness, because like most of us, I didn't realize that I was already innately good and worthy without needing to earn it.

After graduating from high school, I received a scholarship to play soccer at Texas Christian University in Fort Worth, Texas. College was a bit of a lonely and isolating time for me. I excelled on the soccer field and in school, but never really felt like I fit in. I was so focused on keeping up with the rigorous demands of being an athlete and academic that I didn't choose to party or go out much, so I didn't have a whole lot of friends. I pushed myself hard to be the best at everything I did and unfortunately failed to really enjoy the college life.

Straight from college I went to graduate school to get my clinical doctorate degree in physical therapy. I excelled there as well. I enjoyed my time in physical therapy school, learned to lighten up a bit, made some great friends, and met Chad, the man who would eventually become my husband. He says he knew he was going to marry me the day he laid eyes on me. I, on the other hand, did not and it took me a good couple of years to come around. My friends and I would catch him staring at me from across the room and laugh. Eventually, Chad and I became friends and started studying and working out together. He finally got up the nerve to confess his love to me and I turned him down twice (cringe). I was still pretty hung up on a guy I used to date and not open to the idea of a new relationship. Despite the rejection, he just kept on being a consistent and loving presence in my life, and a couple years later we started dating. Chad has always been steadfast in his love and support from the moment I met him. His love has not wavered and has continued throughout the past decade of our life adventure together.

After physical therapy school, Chad and I moved to Austin, Texas. We moved to a new city, got new jobs as physical therapists, studied for our board exams, passed our board exams (whew!), got engaged, and got married, all major life stressors, all within a six-month window. Shortly after our amazing honeymoon to Maui, my health plummeted. Instead of the quintessential post-wedding honeymoon phase of magic and bliss, we went straight to the "in sickness and in health" part of the vows. I know neither of us expected the sickness part would come so soon.

At first a few rashes that looked and felt like poison ivy popped up on my legs. Then I started getting colds more frequently, experiencing joint pain, and was more fatigued than usual. The rashes spread to cover both my legs, my arms, my neck, and my torso. The doctors diagnosed me with "dermatitis," which just means inflammation of the skin, and gave me creams and steroids. They ran my bloodwork and said everything looked "normal." *Do you see my skin?! Do I look normal to you?* I thought. I was getting nowhere, it seemed. I began to feel worse and experience additional symptoms. I was exhausted all the time and started getting headaches and excruciating sinus pain. I didn't want to leave the house because I felt miserable and self-conscious because of the rashes. I didn't want people to stare. I didn't even want people to ask me how I was, because neither the effort of lying and saying I was fine nor telling the truth felt like something I could handle. I felt so isolated and alone. I didn't even want my husband to touch me because my skin hurt so badly and I felt ugly and disgusted by my appearance. This was supposed to be the best time of our lives. We were supposed to be on cloud nine, dreaming about our future and making love in every corner of our new home together. Instead it felt like once Chad and I were married we were dropped into a full-on nightmare. It was such a challenging time for both of us. We felt very isolated and alone. We had no family close by, nor did we have a community to support us.

I was working at a busy physical therapy clinic at the time. I would wear long sleeve shirts and pants to cover up the rashes, even though some of them were visible on my neck and face at times. I had a hard time focusing on my patients who were coming to me to help them with their pain. I tried to listen intently, but the throbbing from my skin grated on my patience and left me feeling so depleted that I had a hard time wanting to help anyone. I came home every day irritable and exhausted. My relationship with Chad was struggling. This whole experience since we said "I do" put a huge strain on our newly budding marriage. The medical bills, the lack of physical intimacy, my inability to work and contribute to the partnership as much as I had before, the fear of me never getting well, the overwhelm, the grief, the anger, and the impossible decisions hung over us like a black cloud. All of this, combined with the typical challenges and growing pains of learning to live with each other and be married was almost too much to bear at times.

As I reflect on this time, I am in awe of how we ever made it through. I wouldn't have made it if it weren't for Chad. He never gave up on me and he never gave up on us. Chad was and is my rock, my love, and I am beyond grateful for his unconditional love and support (which has continued to grow and deepen over ten years of marriage and many challenges, twists, and turns).

I worked until I got so sick that I couldn't anymore and went on short-term disability. This is when I developed the systemic infection and pus-filled lesions in my mouth and throat that I described earlier. Things kept getting worse and my health was in a full-blown downward spiral to the point I wasn't sure if I'd be around much longer. Doctors couldn't figure out what was wrong with me and the drugs weren't working. I tried four different rounds of antibiotics in an attempt to knock out the infection, but the symptoms kept coming back with a vengeance. My doctor was concerned that the infection would spread into my bloodstream. I thought and felt like I might die, and as I mentioned, I was beginning to welcome the idea if this was how I was going to have to live. And then, after much anguish, loathing, and despair, I surrendered. *Okay God, what am I supposed to do?* I prayed.

There was a time between antibiotics that I felt well enough to get out of the house, so Chad took me to the grocery store to get a few things. As I was standing in the checkout line at Whole Foods, an article headline in the *Well Being Journal* caught my eye. The article was titled, "Natural Solutions to Drug-Resistant Infections." *I certainly have a drug resistance infection*, I thought and started reading the article while I waited. I bought it and finished reading it on the car ride home. The article was talking about several natural plant medicines that have been used to treat life-threatening infections. One of which was wild Mediterranean oregano oil, which had been used to knock out extremely serious infections including malaria in third world countries. I was completely captivated, a little skeptical, but hopeful and desperate to try anything. The article suggested a book to read on the subject. I read it, ordered the twenty-dollar bottle of oregano oil, took it, and within three days the infection was gone. Yup. Crazy, right?! And, it was the first time in years that I had some relief from the rashes on my body. After almost two months of battling the infection, taking extremely strong drugs with horrible side effects under the care of one of the best immune and infection specialists in the country, a few drops of oregano oil (that cost pennies per dose) destroyed the infection in three days. I was in awe (and extremely grateful) at the power of this simple and unassuming plant medicine.

A whole new paradigm of healing opened up for me after my healing with oregano oil. I started to ask more questions – a lot more questions – and behold my passion for natural and holistic healing was birthed. I began to learn about nutrition and natural healing methods and became obsessed with learning about all the ways people healed themselves outside of conventional medicine. Up until this point I had never thought about how the food I ate impacted my health. I drank diet sodas and fat-free cream cheese and bagels and thought I was eating pretty healthy. I was always thin and a high-level athlete and got away with eating tons of sugar and processed food without gaining weight or noticing it affect my ability to perform. I often wonder if I had known what I know now about nutrition if I would've been an even better athlete. I ditched the sugar, fast-food, and processed food and began eating healthy, whole, real food.

During this time, I started to seek out holistic health practitioners because I was not getting any answers from the conventional medical doctors I had been seeing. The drugs they had been offering me made me feel worse and I didn't want to take them anymore. I started working with naturopathic doctors and various alternative medicine practitioners. The naturopathic doctors ran their tests and were now finally coming up with some information that could explain some of my symptoms. The various tests revealed autoimmune issues, low thyroid function, adrenal exhaustion, poor liver function, multiple food and environmental sensitivities, parasites and other infections, Epstein Barr virus, heavy metal toxicity, and hormone imbalances. I started supplement protocols, and was encouraged to slow down and rest, get sunshine, do yoga, ditch gluten and dairy, and eat an organic, healthy diet. And let me tell you, I consumed epic amounts of supplements and tried all kinds of therapies and cleanses. I did start to feel better and was able to return to work, but the progress was slow and frustrating. I had a hard time tolerating all the supplements and even some healthy foods. Although I did experience some improvement, I continued to have chronic fatigue, rashes, headaches, sinus pain, and symptoms of a poor immune system.

I became obsessive about my health. I channeled the same intensity that I had for sports into researching and trying to figure out how to get well again. We spent thousands and thousands of dollars on natural therapies, supplements, and doctors. I read book after book. I bought all organic natural food. I learned all about the toxicity in our food supply, water, air, and environment and how much it was contributing to sickness in our world. I removed all the toxins from our home, including the mold I found lurking in the air ducts. I learned about the importance of healing the gut using food and supplements and gradually started to notice the rashes getting better and better.

After a couple years of working with a several different practitioners and getting marginal results, I found a practitioner who used a type of applied kinesiology, or muscle testing, to tap into my body's own intelligence. He confirmed what the other practitioners said about my body being overwhelmed with toxicity and infections, but that I wasn't making progress very quickly because my body wasn't able to tolerate all the supplements, nor able to address all the issues at once. He was able to identify what my body needed to work on first and we began slowly peeling back layers of the onion. I worked with him for quite a while and he helped me gradually restore my health.

I continued to learn about other aspects of holistic healing and applying them to my life. I began to realize how stress impacts the immune system and how being a perfectionist, Type A personality keeps the body chronically amped up, which leads to disease. I was beginning to realize the necessity of slowing down, resting, playing, and enjoying my life. And to be honest, I didn't know how! I realized that I had been living my entire life to please and get approval from other people and I didn't even know what *I* wanted, what made *me* happy, or how to even slow down to figure it out!

Several years after Chad and I were married and after I had made some significant headway, I was finally strong enough to travel. And the rashes were no more!!! We hadn't been on a vacation since our honeymoon years ago because my immune system was too weak to handle the stress of travel. We planned a yoga vacation in Costa Rica that promised healthy food, pristine nature, yoga, and relaxation. It was extraordinary! People from all over the world gathered together in a circle on the eve of the first night of the vacation, introduced themselves, and shared why they had come to such a place. It was magical and was the first time Chad and I sat in such a sacred and loving container where people shared authentically from their hearts. When it was my turn to share the moment felt monumental. Gratitude filled my heart and tears flowed down my face as I shared, how after years of struggling with my health, Chad and I were here in Costa Rica finally fulfilling my dream. I told them of the vision I had played out so many times in my mind while I laid sick in bed. It was the vision of walking hand in hand with Chad on a beautiful beach, wearing a bikini, free of rashes and enjoying the moment fully. There wasn't a dry eye in the room. After such an intimate round of sharing, we all became fast friends – some of which we are still friends with today.

It was in Costa Rica that I met an amazing woman – Lana. She was there teaching a yoga workshop. I was drawn to her like a moth to a flame. She embodied an ease, elegance, and grace – a sense of being comfortable in her own skin that my soul craved. I asked to speak with her and she obliged. I shared my healing journey with her and talked about how much I wanted to feel vibrant again and how I deeply desired to really love and enjoy my life as we dipped our legs into the infinity pool staring at the breathtaking ocean/jungle view.

"What are your passions? What is it that makes you really happy?" she asked.

I sat for a moment, stunned and silent. "I don't know. I don't know what I love to do," I said. I had been achieving, striving, and doing so much for so long that I never actually stopped to ask myself if I really even enjoyed it or actually wanted to do it. Panic seized my chest. How could I not know what I love to do? It sounded so silly, simple, and juvenile. But, I had no answer.

She looked at me with a loving and compassionate smile. "It's okay," she said. "You will. Have you ever sat still in the silence with yourself?" she asked.

"Huh? What do you mean?" I asked.

She asked me if I ever meditated. I was genuinely confused as to how this related to our previous discussion. I said no and honestly had no clue how this would help me. *What was the point?* I thought. She recommended I give it a shot and told me that it would help me to find myself again. "You are just a little lost right now. You have to be silent to hear the whispers of your heart."

"Okay," I said. "So how do I do it?"

She told me to sit quietly and focus on the in and out flow of my breath.

"Okay, and what else?" I said.

"That's it," she replied.

I was pretty skeptical, but I was open to trying new things. I knew deep down that despite not really loving the idea, it was something I needed to try, especially since I admired Lana and wanted to feel more peaceful and connected to my body like she seemed to be.

So, the next morning I sat out by the pool on a cushion. I set a timer for five minutes. I squirmed and temporarily got distracted by the annoying voices in my head urging me to quit and telling me that it was stupid, but I continued. I returned to my breath and for the first time in a long time felt a smidgen of peace, something I hadn't felt in a really, really, really long time. When I went home I continued the morning practice and began to contemplate and explore myself in deeper ways. I made what I call a joy list, which we will talk more about in Chapter 10. I literally kept a running list of the things that make me joyful and started trying out new things. It was so much fun and quite liberating! I built a square foot garden, I bought a bike, and realized how much I love being in nature. In a way, I was getting to know myself for the first time ever.

My healing journey took a turn into deepening my personal development. I realized ways in which my thoughts, beliefs, and ways of being were holding me back and keeping me from feeling the joy, fulfillment, and peace that I desired. I slowed down. I started letting go of the need to be "perfect" all the time. Six months later I returned to Costa Rica on a solo adventure (the first one in my life!) for a one-month certification in Tao Flow yoga, a fusion of yoga and qi gong. It was an incredible experience that taught me many ancient healing practices. It deepened my personal and spiritual inquiry as well as my meditation practice, and challenged me in many ways. When I returned home, I took courses in nutrition, learned about essential oils, and continued my education about holistic healing. I started to dream again and share those dreams with others. I had a burning desire to feel vibrant and amazing. And one of the other things I desired more than anything on the planet was to be a mother and start a family. So, I continued to work diligently on my health.

Chad and I both became passionate about holistic healing and wellness and soaked up all the information we could. As our definition of health and wellness expanded, we started to feel dissatisfied with our jobs as physical therapists. We were eager to share our newfound knowledge about nutrition and holistic health with our patients, but continued to be reprimanded when we did. "Physical therapists aren't supposed to talk about diet," is what our superiors told us. We became frustrated because we knew we could help many of our patients dealing with chronic pain and illness tremendously by addressing nutrition and lifestyle factors. We realized that we really wanted to work with people in a way that would allow us to help them address all aspects of their health. We began sharing what we had been learning with many people that crossed our paths and eventually started a blog about optimal ways of eating, moving, thinking, and living. The blog turned into an online business and then gradually over time we were able to let go of our jobs as physical therapists and focus on holistic health and the preventative side of healthcare.

After about eight years since the initial health crisis, my health had gradually improved. Although I still dealt with some symptoms, overall I was doing pretty well. My energy was much improved, I returned to being able to lift weights again, was able to travel without getting sick, and continued to dive diligently into learning about holistic healing and incorporating what I learned in an effort to improve my health. I continued to work with a handful of practitioners, did acupuncture, ate an organic, whole food diet, deepened my personal growth work, meditated, and continued to hold the deep, heartfelt desire to have a baby. When my closest friends and family would ask how I was doing and when we were going to start a family, I would tell them, "I think we are getting really close – I'm 90% there."

Chad and I finally decided that it was time to start a family. I had two big dreams. Like I mentioned, one was to have a baby, and the other was to go to Italy. We decided that we would plan an epic trip to Italy and finally, after years of health struggles, start our family. We were beyond excited and I could hardly believe it was actually happening.

Two weeks before the big trip we had friends in town for the weekend and were enjoying an evening of laughter and nourishing conversation. I was getting tired and they wanted to stay up, so I excused myself and started getting ready for bed. I changed into my pajamas and, in the process of removing my shirt, was reminded of the soreness in my shoulders and chest from working out a couple days prior. I massaged my pectoral muscles to ease the soreness and as I poked and prodded in different spots on my right chest area, my fingers surprisingly bumped up against something dense and large behind my nipple. It was about the size of a quarter. Fear reverberated in my body like the sound of a gong and I dropped to my knees. I couldn't breathe. I was having a panic attack. No, no, no, no. I can't do this. I knew it wasn't good, I just knew it. I called for Chad to come. He came and held me while I was shaking and crying, not knowing what was going on. I calmed down enough to tell him what I had found, and he felt it too. He told me not to worry and that we would figure it out. To say I was devastated would be a profound understatement – there are no words to describe the feeling that I felt that night.

We were scheduled to leave for Italy in a week. We thought about cancelling the trip, but agreed to go and take the time to reset and try to enjoy ourselves. We would figure out an action plan when we got home. The trip was bittersweet. I enjoyed the sights, sounds, tastes, and smells of Italy the best I could. We cruised the majestic mountains and waters of Lake Como, we each bought scarves to warm our necks and Italian leather boots in Florence, we meandered the stunning waterways of Venice, soaked up the amazing architecture and history of Rome, reveled in the rolling hillsides and wineries of Tuscany, and marveled at the pastel tapestry of buildings built on the hills overlooking the ocean of the Amalfi coast. It was a dream, except that it was a nightmare. I got lost in the beauty of St. Mark's Basilica and then cried moments later as we walked hand in hand down the cobblestone streets eating our gelato as I remembered the sobering reality of what I was going to face when I got home.

I mourned the fact that we would not be starting our family here. I was angry. *God, hadn't I been through enough?* I worked so diligently, so hard for years and years. We'd spent so much money. I'd become a nutrition practitioner, a yogi, and taken the courses and read the books. I'd dedicated my life to healing so that I could have this baby. What was I missing? Clearly everything I thought I knew, I didn't. I felt defeated.

We arrived home and I knew I needed to figure out what to do. I knew deep down it was cancer and I didn't feel that the conventional path of chemo and radiation was the right path for me. Instead of jumping right into researching what to do or polling trusted friends and practitioners about what I should do, which is what I'd done in the past, I got really still and really quiet. It was very clear to me that I had to take a different approach to my healing than what I had currently been doing. Because, despite everything I had tried, learned, and done, I still had a tumor growing in my breast.

I spent several days meditating and taking walks. *What am I supposed to do?* I asked God. And then I heard what I call the "Divine Whisper": *"If you are going to survive, you are going to have to learn to listen to your heart."* I had not ever heard a response from God with such clarity and precision. I took a deep breath and felt a sense of calm and peace after receiving this direction. And then, in the next breath I felt myself contract and panic. *How do I do that?* I thought. I wasn't sure, but I knew getting really quiet and still was part of it. And I knew that staying in a fearful place was not the answer.

I decided to keep things very quiet, only sharing what was happening with my family and closest friends. I was feeling so much fear and overwhelm that in order to learn to listen to my heart for guidance I knew I needed quiet and space – free from the opinions, ideas, and fears of others. Just a mention of the word "cancer" evokes a fearful energy in most people. I knew that the opinions of others would only cloud my ability to learn to listen to my heart and keep me stuck in fear. If my heart really did have all the answers for my highest good, then I wanted to learn to listen. I just hoped I could learn sooner rather than later.

After several days of stillness and meditation I was finally prompted to reach out to our reverend's wife at church for support. It was strange and didn't make a whole lot of sense to me because I didn't really know her that well. I was a little hesitant, but I made the request anyway since I was in the new business of following my heart and all. A few days later we met in person. During the conversation, I found out that she happened to be friends with a woman who was one of my favorite authors and teachers on the topic of healing and spirituality. She owned the holistic healing center that I almost went to years ago when I was really sick. I was blown away at the synchronicity of it all. She asked if I wanted her to reach out to this friend. I said yes and within days I was on my way to meet her at the clinic she owned a few hours away.

I was a little awestruck at our first meeting because I had read several of her books, one of them being the book that had helped me deepen my faith and recover from being so sick years ago. I told her what was going on and how I was scared, but that I didn't feel that going the conventional medical route was the best option for me. She paused and looked at me for a moment. And out of what I thought was left field she said, "You need to learn to receive." *Huh?* I thought. *I just told you all about the lump in my breast and you want me to learn to receive? Receive what?* It would take me many months of learning, reading, and soul-searching to begin to get what she meant.

She proceeded to explain her program and showed me how she used a topical plant-based salve to pull out cancerous tumors through the skin. My jaw dropped as she flipped from picture to picture of actual tumors that had been removed from people's bodies. It was fascinating. I'd never seen anything like it before. The program also included different modalities of detoxification and supplementation, in addition to the topical salve application, which would require me to live at the clinic for a couple months for daily removal and re-application of the salve. I know it may sound crazy to some, but this felt like the right course of action for me. She recommended I start right away.

I walked to my car and sat inside it contemplating what to do. I asked my heart for direction. I knew this was a *huge* commitment, not only financially, but I'd have to move here, stop working, and choose this unconventional path amongst many other possible conventional and alternative options. I called Chad. I told him about the meeting and that I thought I was being called to come here. I held my breath and shut my eyes after the words came out of my mouth. It seemed like such a big decision. I was overwhelmed at what I was going to have to endure and saddened and afraid by the idea of moving here and being away from him. And without a pause, question, or hesitation, he said, "Okay, we're coming with you." He meant him and our mini Goldendoodle pup, Maya. I still get choked up every time I think of this moment. I love him so fiercely for how he responded. There was no doubt or questioning, just total and complete support. Tears ran down my face. It never occurred to me that he would or could come with me. I felt immediate relief and overwhelming love. I headed home and we began looking for an apartment to rent and packing our stuff. A week later we had moved into a place not too far from the clinic.

I spent two months at the clinic and it was a time of deep spiritual growth for me. I journaled and spent large amounts of time in prayer, meditation, and contemplation. Addressing the spiritual aspect of healing was a big part of the program at the clinic, which is one of the reasons I chose it. I spent time in nature reading books about healing and spirituality. I listened to the lectures being taught at the clinic about the True Nature of God, not from the religion of my childhood, but the loving, merciful, all-knowing, all-encompassing presence that is Love and does not condemn or create disease. I began to challenge my own beliefs about disease, God, my own identity, and life. I learned that healing is about remembering and reclaiming our True Identity as divine beings, and knowing that we are already whole and complete. Healing is about choosing to receive the Love of God, not by human effort, which is and has always has been available and never withheld. I soaked up these spiritual teachings and they swirled inside me as I struggled to get out of my head and know them in my heart.

I attended the clinic daily, which was nestled on a piece of beautiful land with trees and a river running through it. I did various treatments that included colonics, juicing, and coffee enemas. I did what we called "the patch" treatment every day, which consisted of the topical salve to pull the cancer out through the skin. It was one of the most painful experiences of my life. Over the course of two months, I watched as gray cancerous matter came out of my breast in the area where I originally felt the mass, as well as all around the axillary or armpit area. There was so much inflammation and swelling that it was hard to tell right away if the mass was gone. Once the swelling went down and it began to heal, we realized there was still a lump behind the nipple area. I was completely devastated. I was grateful that some of the cancer had come out, but why didn't all of it come out? They didn't know, but recommended I go get a biopsy to make sure that what was left was still cancer.

I agreed to see a medical doctor to get the biopsy, but was dreading the appointment. The biopsy was a horrible experience. The doctor was out-raged by the fact that I had deviated from the standard of care and instead opted for this alternative treatment she had not heard of. Her words were harsh, accusatory, and disrespectful, which only amplified the fear I was experiencing. Chad and I left feeling angry and disappointed at the care we received.

We returned a week or so later to get the results. I remember walking into the cancer center feeling chilled, yet sweating through my shirt. The fear and heaviness of the place was palpable and added to my trepidation. Chad and I waited for the doctor to come in for the results. It felt like a lifetime of waiting. Finally, she came in, sat down, and told us the results were positive for cancer. Time stood still and we were both stunned. I was hoping that the mass that was still left was benign since it hadn't pulled out through the skin with the salve treatment. I didn't say anything. I just stared at Chad and he stared back. She abrasively told me I needed to schedule a mammogram and start chemo and radiation right away. She told us she would meet with the tumor board and come up with a specific plan. "Are you going to schedule the mammogram tomorrow?" she repeated, this time with her face about two feet from my face while I started straight ahead.

I turned my head very slowly to look at her in the eyes. "I need to breathe," I said in a very assertive tone. She backed away and relented a bit with the forcefulness of her questions and demands. The silence was thick and no one said a word for what seemed an eternity. "I'm not going to schedule anything right now. I need to go home and feel into what to do next. Thank you." We got up and left and never went back to her. The way she spoke to me in a bullying and fear-based manner was unacceptable.

What do I do now? God, am I hearing you right? Did I make the right choice to go get treatment at that clinic? Why couldn't the whole tumor have come out? I did not know. But I continued my commitment to listen to my heart.

I took a few days to prayerfully contemplate what to do next. At 3 a.m. one very early morning, I woke up and was prompted to get on the computer and type in "holistic breast cancer treatment." I found a holistic breast cancer doctor named Dr. Véronique Desaulniers, or Dr. V for short. She previously went through breast cancer herself and treated it naturally, and was familiar with the topical salve treatment I had used. I resonated with her holistic approach and kind demeanor and started working with her. I loved her immediately. She did several highly-specialized tests and then I started an intensive supplement and holistic healing regimen. Since I was working with her long-distance, she recommended considering going to one of the few alternative cancer clinics in the country that offered some more aggressive treatments. I looked into various clinics and found one in California that had several of the therapies Dr. V recommended. Within a couple of weeks I had a long-distance appointment with one of the doctors. After the appointment, Chad and I prayed about it, talked it through, and decided to go for it. Going to California would mean, once again, picking up our lives and moving elsewhere for a couple months.

But, before I left, I was outside in the backyard and got the nudge to seek out a breast cancer surgeon who was open-minded and supportive – just in case. It surprised me actually, but I followed through. In my mind, I was open to the idea of having surgery if I absolutely felt I needed it, but I did not want to have to go that route. I found a really kind and professional female surgeon who I really liked. I told her about what I had done so far and she was respectful, supportive, open, and curious about the path I was taking. I told her of my plans to go to California. She recommended the surgery right away, but said she understood and advised me not to wait any longer than three months.

Chad and I packed our car and headed to California with Maya in tow to live there for two more months of intensive alternative therapies. The hope was that the tumor would shrink enough that I would be a candidate for highly specialized and non-invasive surgery that would freeze the tumor. A little more than halfway through my treatment we realized that we were running out of money and had depleted our savings. Everything was out of pocket and none of it was covered by insurance. We ended up having to sell our home back in Texas from California to pay for the treatment. Chad's parents and a realtor friend of ours helped us sell our home in one weekend. We were grateful for the money, but I felt a huge sense of guilt and sadness that we no longer had a home to go back to. It was an extremely challenging time for Chad and me. I was no longer working, Chad was working from our rented apartment while I went into the clinic every weekday, and we were spending massive amounts of money on treatments we hoped would save my life. Our online business was on shaky ground and it was a time of intense emotional turmoil and uncertainty.

After two months of treatments I felt great. We did an MRI to see if the tumor had shrunk. It did not. We were devastated again. My doctors there, as well as Dr. V, recommended a mastectomy. I didn't want to do it. I *really* didn't want to do it. After getting the news, I needed space and I needed nature. Chad took me to a park nearby. We got out of the car and the park was full of gorgeous trees with purple blossoms. It felt good to be away from the clinic and I felt like I could breathe again. I took my yoga mat and laid it down in front of one of the trees. I was drawn to it because it was different from the rest. It started to grow upwards like all trees do, but then the trunk took a sharp right turn and was growing sideways. Its branches were covered in purple blossoms and it was beautiful to me. I sat and stared at it. *God, why is this happening to me? Am I not hearing you right? I've done all the things. I went where I thought you wanted me to go. Why isn't the tumor shrinking? You know they want me to do the mastectomy, and we talked about this, I definitely don't want to do that.* I sat in the silence and stared at the tree some more. And this is what I heard.

"She's lopsided but she's still beautiful."

Excuse me, I thought. *What does that mean?* And then it sunk in. *Oh, no, no, no. You're telling me to get the surgery, aren't you? You know I don't want to do it. I don't like hospitals or surgeries. And plus, I'd like to keep both breasts.* I had already thought about the possibility of surgery prior to coming to California. I decided if I were ever to get a mastectomy that I would not get reconstruction. I didn't want to have any foreign materials in my body since I had been so highly sensitive to things like that in the past. God was speaking to me through the tree. Being lopsided wouldn't mean I was any less beautiful, God assured me, but it didn't change the fact that I did *not* want to do the surgery. I needed some time to let this sink in.

We packed up and headed back home to Texas to meet with the surgeon I had found before I left for my second two-month adventure. She did an ultrasound and said that the tumor was pressed up against the pectoral wall and that if it infiltrated the muscle that I would not be a candidate for surgery. She said I needed to move quickly. I knew that removing the tumor wasn't going to completely cure me. I was not getting to the underlying reason why the tumor grew in the first place, but it was going to buy me some time to do the deeper work I knew I needed to do.

I wonder if on some level I knew I would have the surgery, which is why I decided to see a surgeon out of the blue before I left. I could argue that maybe I was "wrong" to go to California because the treatment didn't shrink the tumor, but I know that is not the case. Even though the treatment didn't "work" in the way I had hoped, there were several poignant moments and learnings that happened while I was there. There are always reasons we know not of. It was in California that I really began to hone my ability to listen to my intuition and started noticing how much Spirit was constantly speaking to me through signs, symbols, and synchronicities, if only I was open to receive them. It was as I spent hours walking on Laguna Beach, collecting sea glass, and staring at the ocean most days after treatments that I really began to connect with my heart and love myself. I didn't regret the experience.

Once we returned home, with the help of our amazing friends and family, we packed up our home in a couple days and moved most of it to storage. Chad's parents graciously offered to let us to stay in their second home, a little condo on the lake about forty-five minutes from where we lived. Chad and I are beyond grateful and so in awe of how we were so graciously provided for throughout this journey. I remember sitting with Chad, holding hands on the back porch of our house one last time before we moved out. We cried, said goodbye to our first house we had bought together, reminisced, and savored the moment before we were off for the next chapter of our lives. I was so grateful for the man sitting next to me. Tears flowed like rivers down my face at the love I felt for him for sticking with me and being so willing to give up everything for me. Not once did he say anything or do anything to make me feel bad about having lost our money and our home. With my head on his shoulder and our hands intertwined, we talked and laughed about how it was kind of exhilarating and freeing to have lost everything. We had no choice but to surrender, walk in faith, and lean into grace.

A week later I had the surgery. I told my surgeon I did not want her to remove any of the lymph nodes beyond the couple that they typically remove to detect whether the cancer had spread. It's standard procedure to remove the "sentinel node or nodes," test them during surgery for the presence of cancer, and then proceed to remove more nodes if necessary. My intuition told me not to have her remove any more regardless of the results. She had never had anyone request that, but she agreed.

The surgery was a success. I brought all my essential oils and natural remedies to the hospital and didn't need to use the pain meds beyond the first night. My mom flew in from Colorado and helped care for me before and after the surgery. I healed very quickly with no set-backs. The results from the lymph node biopsy came back, indicating there was no metastasis to the lymph nodes. We were so grateful! The salve treatment had pulled out cancerous masses all around the armpit area and I have no doubt that this, plus all the other treatments, kept the cancer from spreading. The oncologist did not recommend any chemo or radiation, but did recommend that I take Tamoxifen. When I researched the drug, I realized that it had pretty severe side effects that included more aggressive cancer. I told the doctor about my research and that I was choosing not to take it. Surprisingly, he told me that he understood and respected my decision.

I spent the next several months recovering at my in-law's lake condo surrounded by nature. It could not have been a better place to recover from surgery. It was a very peaceful and beautiful time of deep, deep introspection and healing. For my physical body, I began doing some intensive detoxification work, but I knew that there was some emotional and spiritual healing that I needed to do. I asked God to reveal to me any and all fear, toxicity, or negativity that was blocking me from healing and to help me let it go. It was pretty extraordinary what happened next. The teachers, books, and opportunities that crossed my path were exactly what I needed for my healing.

I began studying *A Course in Miracles* and learned more about my divine nature, the power of forgiveness, and how to cultivate inner peace. I read spiritual and personal growth books, took an art-journaling class, and continued to dive further into my heart. I was beginning to understand what it meant to live a whole-hearted life versus being stuck in my head all the time. I was learning to cultivate more connection, creativity, authenticity, compassion, play, stillness, gratitude, and joy in my life and getting more in tune with my intuition. I was learning to let go of fear, scarcity, perfectionism, and the need for approval. I was learning to let go of all the things that did not serve me and continued to rediscover who I really am. The inner work wasn't always easy (there were many tears and moments of darkness), but what was there for me on the other side was more beautiful and amazing than I could've ever imagined.

During this time, I crossed paths with a healer and spiritual teacher named Dennis who previously had a cancer center in the Amazon jungle. He was well-versed in using indigenous plant medicines from the jungle for deep physical, emotional, and spiritual healing. I decided to join him in Mexico to learn from him and do the deep emotional and spiritual work that I knew I needed to do. This decision changed my life. I spent the next year working with and being mentored by him. I uncovered deep emotional blocks and subconscious beliefs that had been negatively impacting my health and keeping me from experiencing the peace and joy I longed for. I was able to release so much grief, sadness, anger, and resentment during that time. I felt so much fear fall away. I soon began to realize I could tap into my own healing power and consciously create a life that I love through choosing my beliefs, thoughts, feelings, words, and actions and learning to truly love myself. I will forever be grateful to Dennis for his guidance and support.

Over time, Chad and I deepened our connection and our marriage became stronger than ever. We've learned to not "sweat the small stuff" and our lives have taken on a whole new richness and depth than ever before. We saved up enough money to buy a beautiful home surrounded by nature with a view of the lake. Now, we watch the sunrise in the morning from our balcony and go for walks in the evening around the water to see the sunset. We've been able to travel to beautiful places and have had some amazing adventures together. Cancer, amongst many things, has taught me the importance of cultivating connection. I've always deeply desired community, true authentic connection, and a group of friends to do life with. We now have an extraordinary community of friends who are like family and we love them dearly. We have community gatherings in our home and by the lake and our life is overflowing with deep, heartfelt connection, community, laughter, song, dance, and fellowship. Nothing beats doing life in community and being able to share the joys, sorrows, celebrations, and challenges of life with others.

For so many years I could never quite figure out my purpose and it ate at me. The more I tried to figure it out, the more it eluded me. But, now, as I learn to flow with life and live from my heart, I am uncovering my purpose and realizing that sharing my story and empowering, supporting, and inspiring women to heal and to thrive is a big part of it. My greatest fear when I was diagnosed with cancer was that I would die having never fully lived. Now, I am finally living – like really *living* – and not just sitting on the sidelines of this one and only life I have. I'm traveling, dancing, cultivating community, trying new things, and sometimes falling flat on my face, but learning in the process. I'm growing and stretching, willing to be vulnerable, and finding the authentic version of myself. I'm learning to feel my feelings and love what I feel, to find peace in the uncertainty and perfection in each moment. I'm learning to love myself more and more every day, with all my quirks, scars, beauty, and uniqueness. I'm remembering who I am as a beloved child of God and as a co-creator of my own life experience. I feel so much more fulfillment, connection, peace, wholeness and joy in my life. And for all of this, I am beyond grateful.

Chapter 2:

Whole-Hearted Healing

*"Healing is not creating perfection – there is a Perfect part of us that
is whole – so, we don't heal anything,
we reveal that which is already whole."*
– Ernest Holmes

A Different Way

There is an explosion of chronic disease in our world and it has become among one of the greatest health challenges of the twenty-first century. Many chronic conditions such as cancer, auto-immune disease, and heart disease are being referred to as "diseases of civilization" because they speculate that most chronic diseases stem from modern living – the way we eat, move, think, and live. One article review of cancer states that, "Only 5–10% of all cancer cases can be attributed to genetic defects, whereas the remaining 90–95% have their roots in the environment and lifestyle."[1]

The good news in all of this is that we have *way* more control over our health than we realize. It's time to take that power back and that's what the Whole-Hearted Healing approach and the 9 Essentials are all about. We've been fighting and waging war on cancer and various diseases, yet we still continue to be one of the most chronically sick, medicated, anxious, lonely, depressed, addicted, disconnected, and obese civilizations of all time. If science and experts are pointing to the environment and how we are living as the biggest culprits in chronic disease, and we are continuing to get sicker and unhappier, then it's time to stop and look at what's going on and perhaps try a different way.

I, too, realized that after eight years of spinning my wheels and "fighting" for my health, I needed to find a different way. Finding a cancerous tumor in my breast after all the effort, time, money, and attempts I made to heal myself, there was nothing left to do but surrender and plead to God for help. It was the "Divine Whisper" that I mentioned in the last chapter, that coaxed me into a different way of living and looking at my life and my health. I call this different way Whole-Hearted Healing, which is essentially a holistic, heart-centered way of living. After so desperately and exhaustively seeking and searching outside myself for the answers, I was invited to go within and "listen to my heart." To me this was revolutionary and completely foreign. Like most people, I was never taught how to listen to my heart and I didn't really know what that meant or how to do it, but I made a full commitment to God and myself to learn.

My whole-hearted journey has had its twists, turns, plenty of tears, and challenges, but has been nothing short of exquisite. Exquisite means "extremely beautiful and intensely felt" … and is the best way I've found to put this experience into words. It was the following of my heart and learning to love myself and my life that allowed for true healing to take place. Ironically, it was the opposite of forcing, desperately seeking, and fighting for my health, which I was so accustomed to, that cracked me open to allow healing to unfold. It was a different way of living and approaching my health indeed. The fear that gripped my heart and the frenzied way I approached life gradually began to fall away and I began to learn to listen to my intuition, trust the divinity within me, walk in faith, and flow with life. And to my surprise, my heart led me to an experience of healing and wholeness that I tried so long and hard to find. I came to experience more peace, love, connection, freedom, and joy – all the things I had been chasing my whole life.

If you are reading this and have been struggling, fighting, and trying to figure out your health, but you continue to come up short, disappointed, frustrated, and even miserable, I invite you to open to a new way of approaching your health and life. The ever-expanding lists of diagnoses and dismal statistics on the prevalence of chronic disease, as well as the overwhelming number of people dissatisfied and unhappy with their lives is indicative that we must stop doing the same things and expecting different results. I truly believe that disease can be a divine opportunity for you to wake up and remember who you really are and experience the love, peace, and joy that you crave (and deserve) but haven't been able to find.

The Power Within

If one woman gets – I mean, *really* gets – this one thing from reading my book, then it will make all the time and energy and resources spent writing and publishing this book worth it. You, my love, have the power inside of you to heal. It's not out there. It's inside. I know this is radically contrary to what we were told to believe. We were led to believe that we need to be fixed, saved, and that we are not enough as we are. You are enough, and in fact, you are powerful beyond measure. I remember when I was first told this, it was hard to believe, but somewhere deep inside I knew it was Truth and I knew it was the path to healing and reclaiming my wholeness.

The truth is this – the power that created the cosmos, turns embryos into babies, keeps your heart beating, and turns acorns into oak trees is the power that created you and is the power that can heal you. Your body was created by Divine Intelligence (i.e. God) and is always moving toward a state of balance and wholeness. It's your job to let go of the fear, interferences, and all things blocking you from Love and that state of wholeness (which you will learn more about in this book). You actually are a magnificent expression of this Infinite Power and it resides inside you. It is my hope that by reading this book, and planting this seed in your consciousness, that this Truth will trickle down from your head to your heart to your knowing.

What Does It Mean to Be Healed?

I chased, sought, prayed, wished, and longed to be healed for a decade. I wanted my physical symptoms to go away, but there was more. I wanted to feel whole – to feel at peace, alive, joyful, connected, loved, fulfilled, comfortable in my own skin, and free. I wanted to love my life. And likely deep down that's what you desire and it's what you deserve. We all do.

I've been fascinated, and maybe a little obsessed, with the topic of healing ever since I got sick years ago. I've often contemplated and pondered many questions about healing: *What does it mean to be healed? Where does healing come from? How do we heal? And why do some people heal and others do not?*

A poignant conversation with Dennis, my spiritual teacher from the jungle I mentioned last chapter, really helped me to understand the true nature of healing. Before I decided to work with Dennis I wanted to speak with him in person. I asked him if he thought these plant medicines he worked with and knew so much about could heal me. He paused, took a breath, and said he wanted to tell me two stories. "Okay," I said and listened intently.

Story 1: He told me of a woman with breast cancer that came to his cancer clinic many years ago. She had several tumors in her breasts. She stayed at the clinic for many months and participated in the program, which consisted of many things including juicing and consuming indigenous plant medicines. She cleansed her body, worked through deep emotional blockages, had huge breakthroughs, and began to feel a deeper sense of peace and love in her life. After several months, she left the clinic and returned to her doctors back home. She found out that her tumors were gone and went on to live a life of much more love, fulfillment, ease, and joy than before her time in the jungle.

Story 2: Another woman arrived at the clinic with Stage 4 cancer of some kind and was in poor shape physically – as well as mentally, emotionally, and spiritually. She was an angry and resentful woman, was estranged from her family, and had a tumultuous relationship with her husband. She participated in the program and began to heal her pain and sorrow. The woman reconnected with her husband and he eventually joined her there at the clinic. They rekindled their romance and learned to love each other again. She also reconnected with her family, with whom she hadn't spoken in years. They too, came to be with her in the jungle. She released the bitterness and resentment that she had harbored for so long, she forgave, and she surrendered. Her body continued to shut down, but she came to know deep peace, had returned love to her life, and she passed away surrounded by her loved ones.

"Both women were healed," he told me.

Yes. I had tears in my eyes and a warmth in my chest, because I knew the truth of this rang so completely in my being. Healing is about so much more than the disappearance of symptoms from the physical body. Something shifted in me after hearing these stories and I began to contemplate life and death differently and look underneath the fear I had of dying.

We don't talk about it much, but death is inevitable. Our physical bodies will one day – whether tomorrow, three months from now, or forty years from now be no more. No one gets a hall pass on this one. We're all going to die. I really let this sink in for a moment in a way I hadn't before. And then it hit me. I realized my fear of dying was blocking me from truly living and healing. I had been praying for God to remove all the blockages to me knowing my True Nature and trusting in my innate ability to heal – this fear of dying was a big one.

Yes … I was afraid to die. And the thought of dying now, at such a young age (in my thirties), made me feel like a failure. The thought surprised me. *At what age would dying no longer make me a failure?* I questioned. *Was it sixty or seventy or eighty or ninety? Just because a woman lives to ninety or one hundred years old, does that make her "successful" or better than someone who dies at forty? What if the woman who dies at ninety has lived a miserable life – angry, lonely, and estranged from her family and friends? Would I rather live into my nineties and be miserable versus dying at forty having lived a life of love, connection, meaningful experiences, and fulfillment?* Of course not. Interesting.

What I realized is that underneath my fear of dying was *actually* this: I was afraid to die without ever having fully lived. I was in my thirties and felt like I had wasted so much time being afraid and tiptoeing through life. Like so many, I was afraid of living, afraid of dying, afraid of failing, afraid of never figuring it out, afraid of not being enough, and ultimately afraid of my greatness. I was living a life of quiet desperation, trying to fit in, hoping to be a "success," trying not to let anyone down, and keeping my light hidden. I had yet to really go for my dreams or even give myself permission to *really* thrive. I had yet to fully share my gifts with the world, find my "purpose," be a mother, or have the epic adventures and experiences I desired to have. I had been "trying really hard" and "doing all the right things" that successful people do in life, like get lots of degrees, get scholarships to reputable universities, and get married – but I wasn't truly happy, fulfilled, able to express myself the way I wanted, or comfortable speaking my truth, nor was I being the full authentic *me* that I longed to be. I wasn't living. I was hiding. The enormity of this realization, although a profound gift, caused me to feel an immense amount of grief for the time that (I judged in that moment) had not been lived whole-heartedly.

There is a quote by Oliver Wendell Holmes that says, "Many people die with their music still in them. Too often it is because they are always getting ready to live. Before they know it, time runs out." Now faced with the possibility of death, I realized I had mostly been hanging out on the sidelines of my life warming up for the big game, but never feeling ready or confident enough to get on the court. I couldn't believe it. Why am I just realizing this now? I didn't want to die with my music still inside me – I had entire symphonies to share with the world.

Some of you reading this will resonate with what I've just shared. You are afraid to die "too soon" or "too young" or die without fully *living*. Or maybe you're putting your life on hold waiting to fully recover or rid yourself of the symptoms that you are experiencing, waiting for that "one day" when things will be perfect. Maybe you're afraid you won't ever overcome your current circumstances, which keeps you in a holding pattern of sadness and regret. I can relate to feeling and thinking all of these things. But, it's the very fear we hold in our minds and bodies about death and life as we know it, as well as the resistance and unwillingness to accept our current circumstance as it is that keeps us from healing, fully living, experiencing wholeness and the possibility of what it means to thrive.

I remember sitting in front of my dear friend and mentor, Fran, (who is also an incredible healer) and processing with her my feelings of overwhelming grief, fear, and sadness during the time I was dealing with breast cancer.

"Tell me what you are afraid of," she asked.

"I'm afraid I'll never be a mom," I said as tears pierced the corners of my eyes and streamed down my face dripping off my chin. "I've wanted to be a mom my whole life. I've been married for eight years and we haven't conceived because of all the health challenges I've had to deal with. Now, I'm scared I'll never get the chance to have a child of my own." I said unable to hold back the sobs.

Fran looked at me lovingly and never in the way that people do when they feel sorry for you. That's one thing I love most about Fran. "What are the feelings you think you will feel when you are a mom that you most desire to feel?" she asked.

She caught me off guard with her question and I stopped crying and paused to reflect. "Well … I would feel unconditional love, intimate connection, adoration, and be able to nurture, care, teach, and learn from my child."

And what she said next changed my life forever. She smiled and said, "Cultivate that now." Something shifted inside me. I left with the resolve to begin finding ways to cultivate those feelings more intentionally in my life. I started a women's circle in which I was able to experience profound connection, love, and able to nurture and be nurtured in ways that I deeply longed for. I put her advice into practice and the fear of not being a mother started to gradually dissolve.

So, what is the antidote to being afraid to die, having never fully lived? Fully live *now*! I realized staying stuck in the past wishing it could have been different or waiting for "one day" when life is perfect would not serve me and only perpetuated my fear and angst. I started to get on the court of my life. I let my music out. I began living and loving fully from my heart. I started cultivating the feelings and life I wanted to experience. I watched my life magically explode into a flurry of dance, song, passion, adventure, deep connection, community, meaning, fulfillment, wholeness, and LOVE. I began to live the life I always imagined and my physical health improved without me focusing and obsessing about it so much. I experienced healing – in heart, soul, mind, and body. And you can too. The 9 Essentials in this book are your roadmap to healing and living fully *now*.

So, is healing strictly about keeping the physical body alive and free of pain and fully functional? While that may be part of it, it is by no means the whole enchilada. And although we often approach healing in this way, I don't believe it will ever translate into the experience of what we deeply desire at our core, which is peace, joy, the truest experience of love and wholeness, and a deep connection to God, others and our true authentic selves. While it's wise to care for our physical bodies it's even more essential to realize the wholeness of our beings – to identify as and care for the spiritual, mental, and emotional aspects of who we are, in addition to the physical.

I love this quote from Sue Sikking in her book *Beyond Miracle*:

"Healing is not simply the result of a sick body made well. Wholeness and healing are a state of being, the result of knowing who and what we are."

Letting Go

In order to know who and what we are and experience wholeness, we have to let go of who and what we are not. For me, chronic illness and especially cancer became the catalyst to dive deep into my being, and begin to unearth and let go of all that wasn't aligned with Love and Truth and the life I dreamed of having. It was an opportunity to step into more peace, love, and fulfillment than I had ever experienced. I've learned that the process of healing, of awakening to my True Nature, is an emptying and an unraveling. It's the opening of clenched fists and a guarded heart. It's transitioning from fear to love, rigidity to expansion, rehearsed to real, striving to allowing, and forcing to flowing.

Ultimately healing isn't so much about fixing what is broken or gaining something outside of yourself, it's about letting go of all that isn't the deep down divine *you*. It's about letting go of the accumulation of limiting thoughts and beliefs, suppressed emotions, false identities, fear, and toxic foods, habits, relationships, etc. – all of which does not affirm life and the vibrant health you desire. Essentially, it's about letting go of the old accumulation of toxic buildup in body, mind, heart, and soul to reveal the whole, well version of yourself that has been there all along.

Wholeness and Spiritual Identity

"Healing" comes from an Anglo-Saxon word that means "restore to whole." Essentially, when we truly heal we restore our wholeness – which is our natural state and one that we don't have to go find, but one that we remember and return to. Robert Brumet, author of *A Quest for Wholeness*, states that wholeness is a paradox because it is our journey *and* our destination. As spiritual beings, we are already whole and in our humanness wholeness is that which we desire to experience and return to.

Both women in the jungle story told by Dennis experienced healing because they experienced a return to wholeness. Wholeness can be defined many different ways, by many different people, but to me it is an experience of "being well in my soul," knowing my true identity as a piece of the Divine in expression and having the sense of feeling connected to all of Life. Sikking described it as a "state of being" and a "result of knowing who and what we are." It is what our soul craves and is what all the internal clamor and dissatisfaction and disease is nudging us back to. Wholeness is about moving from self-sufficiency to spiritual dependency and realizing we are spiritual beings at our core.

Mother Theresa used the term "spiritual deprivation" when referring to the biggest problem facing the world today. We are completely disconnected from the Divine within us and each other. We think and feel we are separate and that we have to figure everything out on our own. We work so hard to earn love and worthiness, but the Truth is that we already are that which we are seeking. It is the inherited faulty mental programs, beliefs, and constructs about who we are and who God is, that create a state of disease, disconnection, and dissatisfaction within our lives. As you move forward through the 9 Essentials in this book, began to shift your identity as being solely your physical nature to knowing yourself as Spirit in a human body. In doing so you will begin to align with your innate power within to heal.

Our Four Bodies

In addition to being a spiritual being at your core, you have three other "bodies" or aspects of who you are. You have a physical body of course, but also an emotional and mental body. As you already know, your physical body is made up of your bones, muscles, organs, and glands and is the vehicle you use to experience this life. Your emotional body is your feeling system that manufactures love and fear-based emotions. Emotions provide texture and richness to your life. Your mental body is your intellect or thinking mind. It is essential for helping you function in this world. It helps you solve problems, strategize, and make choices. Each are essential components to who you are and you must take into account all four of these bodies in order to truly heal and experience being well and whole.

Holistic (Whole-istic) Health

I want to take a moment to talk about the distinction between a holistic approach and the conventional medical approach to health and healing. A holistic approach looks at the whole person and how she relates to her environment. Instead of focusing on managing disease or isolating body parts or systems, this approach takes into account the interrelatedness of the physical, emotional, mental, and spiritual aspects of a human being. The focus is on helping people experience their maximum potential and well-being in all areas of life.

Conversely, the conventional medical model views health as the absence of disease. We know that health is about much, much more than that! It fails to look at the wholeness of a person and focuses on treating physical symptoms versus getting to the underlying or root of the problem. Any effort you make to improve your health or plan of action you take to heal, that fails to take into account the wholeness of who you are, will likely fall short in some way and may never get you the results you truly desire. This is especially the case with chronic symptoms and chronic illness.

Conventional medicine has its place and excels in emergency medicine and necessary surgeries, but often falls short when used as the *only* tool when it comes to chronic illness. It may end up being a valuable resource as part of your healing path, however I recommend you use it while still taking a holistic and integrated approach to your health. For example, I ended up having surgery during my cancer journey because my intuition guided me to do so. But, I also knew that just cutting out a tumor did not get to the root or underlying reason why it was there in the first place. In addition to the surgery, I also incorporated the 9 Essentials in this book and focused on things like healing emotional wounds, as well as detoxification of my physical body and incorporating many of the lifestyle factors you will learn about in Chapter 7. Be wary of relying totally on conventional medicine to "fix" you. Not only is this giving your power away, which we will talk about in Chapter 3, but this approach to healing is very narrow and limited in its approach and view of health.

As an example, let's look at the difference between taking a holistic approach versus a strictly conventional approach to dealing with heartburn. Lately, you've been experiencing more and more frequent heart burn. You keep taking an antacid every time you feel it and it helps it go away, but it keeps coming back and you aren't sure why. You go to the doctor and she puts you on something stronger, acid reflux medication, to suppress the acid that she says is causing the pain. You start taking it and you are so excited because you haven't felt the burning in weeks. A few weeks go by and although the acid reflux is gone, you realize you are also having headaches and trouble sleeping. *Where's that coming from?* you wonder. You pop an ibuprofen and some sleeping pills. Problem solved – at least for the time being. When you don't take the ibuprofen or sleeping pills the headaches return and you can't sleep. So – you keep taking them because you have a huge trial coming up and you are the lead prosecutor on a case that is going to provide the much-needed money to pay for your children's braces.

You don't realize that by taking the acid reflux medication to suppress the stomach acid, you are not addressing the underlying cause as to why acid is coming up into your esophagus, and you may actually be setting yourself for some serious health issues. Chronic suppression of stomach acid with acid reflux medication can lead to issues with bacterial overgrowth, issues with nutrient absorption, impaired resistance to infection, and could set you up for increased risk of cancer, digestive problems, and other health issues.[2] Acid reflux medication also has a laundry list of side effects, including headaches. Who knows if the headaches and sleeplessness are coming from the drug or the fact that you are feeling a lot of stress lately?

Taking drugs to suppress symptoms, as well as the side effects from the drugs, can create a cascade of imbalance and disharmony in the body, causing more and more symptoms now or days, months, and years down the line. It sets you up for chronic disease. What if you had the self-awareness and emotional intelligence to ask yourself, "*Why do*

I keep having this acid reflux, headaches, and sleeplessness?" and sat still and listened to your answer? You would've realized that the acid reflux popped up every time you've been stressed from working on this particular case, which usually causes you to end up getting fast food, which you typically don't eat. You realize that the food may have something to do with it. You also check in with how you are feeling and realize you are feeling a significant amount of stress and fear. You're afraid that if you blow this case that you won't be able to pay for all the bills that keep piling up and go so far into debt that you won't be able to get out. You're worried you aren't a good mom if you can't buy your daughter those braces and start saving for college. Just bringing awareness to these thoughts, breathing into your heart, feeling the fear, and allowing it to move through you makes your head stop throbbing. You stop to ask your heart for help. What do you need to do to deal with this? You have tools in your tool kit for dealing with stress and you are guided to use them. You decide to resume your morning meditation practice to reduce stress and you make plans to get up thirty minutes earlier tomorrow. You make a decision to prep food at night to bring to work so you don't eat food you know isn't good for you, plus you'll have some time to exercise before lunch since you don't have to go pick anything up, which always helps you feel better.

You are on alert for those icky, grimy thoughts about you "not being good enough" and "being a failure," and you are able to notice them without getting swept up in the negativity. You say your affirmations aloud and make a point to take mini breathing breaks at work. The acid reflux, headaches, and sleeplessness go away within a week. No need for antacids or acid reflux medication or ibuprofen or the sleep medication and the potential disastrous side effects. This is an example of symptoms in the physical body that came from poor diet and mental/emotional stress. When you addressed the issue from a holistic perspective, you were able to heal without going down the rabbit hole of medications, dangerous side effects, and potentially long-term health implications and imbalances.

As you navigate your healing journey, I invite you to take a holistic or "whole" body approach to healing and use conventional medicine as needed and guided to do so. Sometimes symptoms are super intense and a drug or surgery is helpful or necessary and that's okay. Conventional medicine can be very helpful at times. As always, do what you feel called to do and use your intuition, but realize that the cessation of symptoms isn't necessarily the whole story. Avoid thinking that *only* treating symptoms is what is going to truly get you well.

All about the Heart – It's Not Woo-Woo, I Promise

When some people hear things like "listen and live from the heart" they think it's a bunch of woo-woo mumbo-jumbo. I assure you it is not. Once I made the intention to live from my heart, I was blown away to find out that there is actually science that explains the benefits of doing so and corroborates what ancient cultures recognized long ago about the heart's wisdom. For the past twenty to thirty years, scientists and organizations, such as the HeartMath Institute, have discovered extraordinary information about the intelligence and power of the heart, which, when accessed, can help us heal and live more peaceful and fulfilling lives.

The heart is much, much more than a muscle that pumps blood to our entire body and keeps our physical body alive. The heart, just like the mind, has its own governing ability, but is actually more powerful! The heart is over one hundred times more powerful magnetically and is sixty times more powerful electrically than the brain, (as measured using an electrocardiogram.)[3] The electromagnetic field of the heart actually extends out several feet in circumference around the body, allowing the energy and messages from our heart to affect those around us and vice versa.

The heart is incredible – it's a complex organ that has its own "heart-brain," nervous system, and intelligence that can harmonize the systems of the body allowing us to experience greater overall health and well-being. The heart even starts beating in a developing fetus before the brain is formed! Amazing, right?! The heart and brain are constantly communicating. The heart communicates with the brain through various forms of communication (neurological, biophysical, biochemical, and electromagnetic) and actually sends more information to the brain than the brain does to the heart.

When the brain and heart are in sync and working together, we experience a state of harmony, optimal physiological functioning, and well-being. In this state, we are able to reduce stress and anxiety, improve our ability to access our intuition and be more present and resilient in response to the challenges of life. These are all key elements when it comes to healing! This optimal state is called heart coherence and is something we can learn to do on our own and reap the benefits of in our daily life. We will talk more about heart coherence in Chapter 6.

Cultivating Qualities of the Heart

During my Whole-Hearted Healing journey and while taking my commitment to learn to listen and live from my heart seriously, two sources of information that were instrumental in my learning to access my heart made their way into my hands. One was Brené Brown's book *The Gifts of Imperfection*. In it she shares ten guideposts for whole-hearted living that she found during her research on men and women who were living deep, meaningful, and happy lives – which she called "whole-hearted living." The other source was the HeartMath Institute, which I've mentioned. Through these sources I began to realize that cultivating qualities of the heart into my everyday life experience was essential in being able to access and live from my heart.

These heart qualities included: courage, compassion toward myself and others, connection, forgiveness, gratitude, joy, love, non-judgment, authenticity, vulnerability, play, rest, laughter, and kindness. Implementing these qualities intentionally into my life was revolutionary and life-changing and infused it with so much richness, fulfillment, and meaning. I noticed that I was happier and more peaceful. And when you are happy, more at peace, and more content you put your body in a state that is much more conducive to healing. A happy heart is essential to a happy body and immune system! Cultivating the qualities of the heart into your life is another important component of what I call Whole-Hearted Healing. We will talk more about cultivating gratitude, joy, forgiveness, stillness/rest, play, and connection in the pages that follow.

So many women on a healing journey, including myself, think "when I get better" or "when I heal" they will have more fun, play more, be more fulfilled, have better relationships, help others, or do the things they dream of doing or feel the way they dream of feeling. The irony is that when you cultivate the qualities of the heart, as well as take action on the desires of your heart *now* – that is exactly what helps your body heal. Live fully from your heart *now*!

The Heart vs. the Head

Typically, we allow the head to run the show and get completely disconnected from our hearts and this is where we get in trouble. We are taught *a lot* about intellectual intelligence, but not much about how to access the intelligence of the heart or our intuition. The brain is very important in making decisions, strategizing, reading, writing, talking, and helping us function in this world. It's absolutely necessary! However, when we stay "stuck in our heads" or ruled by the "ego mind" without being informed by our hearts, we live in a fearful state and often spend most of our time experiencing depleting emotions, such as anger, fear, and worry. We will talk more in later chapters about how chronic stress and fear create disease in the body.

There is a saying, "the mind is a wonderful servant, but a terrible master." This couldn't be any further from the truth! Whole-Hearted Healing is all about letting the heart lead. Learning to lead and make intuitive decisions with your caring and loving heart, and using your mind as a helpful tool to navigate your life, helps you to experience more of what you want in life and helps you shift from fear to love, which is the energy at which you heal.

Let's Begin

I have found that Whole-Hearted Healing – embracing and embodying our wholeness and leading and living from the heart – is the portal or the pathway to true healing. When we remember who we are as spiritual, emotional, physical, and mental beings and we take a whole-istic approach to our health we invite deeper levels of healing, fulfillment and meaning into our lives. Living from the heart helps us to be better at making decisions for our highest good, allows us to naturally experience more peace, love, connection, and joy. It is through accessing and cultivating the qualities of the heart that we enrich our lives, raise our vibration, and awaken our healing power!

This disease or health challenge is a call for you to awaken, dear one. Instead of staying stuck in the paralyzing fear of what may come, see this as your divine opportunity for deeper discovery of who you are and why you are here. See this as a sacred time to come home to your Self and begin to live the life that you've desired but never knew how to experience.

Whole-Hearted Healing is a journey from head to heart, from fear to love, and from forcing to flowing with life. As you navigate your own journey, embrace and honor every part of your path, however it unfolds, for there are no two paths alike. Through the next several chapters we will explore the 9 Essentials that are key components of your holistic healing roadmap, which will help guide you on your unique path to healing and thriving.

Chapter 3:

Essential #1 –
Taking Responsibility for Your Health

"The more you take responsibility for your past and present, the more
you are able to create the future you seek."
– Author Unknown

Stop Giving Your Power Away

I attended a few support group meetings after my mastectomy. Most were quite helpful, however there was one meeting that left me feeling incredibly sad and angry. We each went around and shared our healing journeys. There were many heart-wrenching stories shared and the overall energy of the space was one of disappointment and fear. I felt like leaving, but I stayed any way. I vividly remember one woman in particular, Nadine, who was sitting next to me. She shared that she recently received shocking news that her breast cancer had metastasized and was in the process of creating a will because she was told she wouldn't live much longer. Her anger was palpable, and understandably so. Tears welled up in the corners of her eyes as she talked about all the milestones she would miss in her children's life. "I did everything the doctors said and I'm still dying," she shared. "Ten years ago, I had Stage 1 breast cancer and did the chemo and radiation and took the drugs, and now I'm dying. How could this happen when I did everything they told me to do?" she questioned.

My heart hurt for her – not only because of this recent diagnosis, but also because I could sense she held so much anguish, resentment and fear in her heart. She felt betrayed because she put her faith fully in the doctors and treatments to heal her. She went on for several minutes and began to talk about other women she knew dealing with metastatic cancer and started criticizing their choices. She was clearly speaking from a place of so much hurt and pain. It was uncomfortable for the entire room and the moderator said nothing.

I put a hand on her back, which seemed to snap her out of her momentary outpouring of passionate anger. "I'm sorry Nadine," I said and we all let her cry in silence for a few minutes.

I believe that no matter the severity of the diagnosis, there's always hope and opportunity for healing to transpire. In an attempt to perhaps share some possibilities of alternative treatments she could explore and offer some hope, I asked her if she tried any other healing measures or modalities besides conventional medicine in the past ten years. She said, "No – the doctors told me that chemo, radiation, and the drugs were the only thing I needed to do so that's what I did."

She was so stuck in her anger and resentment that she wasn't in a place to hear anything I had to say. And that's okay. I kept quiet and felt my heart breaking for her. As I drove home from the support group I cried for Nadine. I felt anger that Nadine had not been educated in other treatment options or the importance of taking a holistic approach to her health. I felt sad at the amount of resentment she had inside of her and at how disempowered and hopeless she felt. I prayed she would find peace, healing, wholeness, and acceptance in the midst of her current circumstances. And after uttering that prayer I felt a surge of responsibility to share what I've learned about the importance of taking a holistic approach to healing so that I might possibly provide a roadmap for healing, peace, joy, wholeness, and empowerment to women like Nadine and so many others (including myself) who have ever struggled and suffered because of chronic illness.

So often, like Nadine, we unknowingly give our power away to doctors, healers, pills, and potions – things outside of ourselves – expecting them to fix us, heal us, and to know what is the absolute best for us. I did this for years. We have this cultural mindset that doctors have the supreme authority over our health and lives. By placing all the power and authority in their hands, we give ours away. When you go to see a doctor or healer to get their expert advice, they are working for *you*. Don't be afraid to ask your questions, state your concerns, and understand this is only one person's advice and perspective and don't be afraid to consider getting multiple viewpoints. Know that ultimately, you know what's best for *you*. Learning to listen to your heart and trusting your intuition above all is key when navigating any health challenge.

It's also important to consider that conventional doctors seldom take a holistic approach to healing and focus mainly on treating physical symptoms, which are only a manifestation of an underlying imbalance or disharmony in one or several of the four bodies we talked about in the last chapter. Remember, you are not just a physical body! No matter if you are seeking conventional medical help or taking a natural or alternative approach (or a combination of both), there is no one person or no one thing that will heal you. This mindset will only disempower you, disappoint you, block your ability to access your own innate healing power and intuition, and lead you further away from your ultimate desire to be well. It doesn't mean that you won't seek the guidance of a doctor or healer or utilize a particular treatment or medicine in your healing process. These may be healing tools that you are guided to implement that will help support your own natural healing process. The important thing here is to relinquish the mindset that it's someone else's responsibility to fix or heal you. Take responsibility for your health and life and begin to learn to trust your intuition to guide you and your body's extraordinary ability to heal itself.

The Victim and the Hustler

Two ways I often see women give their power away during their healing journey is by assuming the role of victim or hustler. You won't get the results you truly want by being a victim or a hustler and you will waste a lot – I mean, a *lot* – of energy that could be channeled into healing and creating a life that you really love.

The Victim

When you are in pain, tired, experiencing debilitating symptoms, afraid, and faced with challenging decisions, it's easy to slip into the "why me" victim mode. It's a completely natural and understandable response. However, if you stay stuck here you will have a hard time healing and likely only perpetuate more of the same reality you are currently experiencing. When you get wrapped up in being "the victim," you often blame other people and circumstances for your health problems and begin to think your life is beyond your control. It's so easy to get consumed with self-pity, fear, pessimism, and anger. You may even begin to unknowingly feed off the attention you get from being sick and blame your illness on your job, your childhood, or your genetics. These may be contributing factors, but expending your energy blaming other people or circumstances keeps you stuck.

This is a very slippery slope, because once the victim mindset takes over it's hard to find your way out and you begin to identify with your diagnosis or symptoms. This is one of the worst things you can do. It's important to never own your illness by saying and thinking "my diabetes" or "my cancer" (later, we will discuss how powerful words and thoughts truly are). You may be dealing with diabetes or cancer right now, but it's not your identity. It's so important to remember the Truth of who you are as a child of the Infinite who has within her the ability to heal and be whole. This is your true identity.

Sometimes the symptoms get so fierce and the fear is all-consuming – I know this place well. When and if this happens, or if you are experiencing this as you read these words, I want to share a quote that I kept on a note card pinned to the wall by my bed to read as a daily reminder:

"This is the principle of LIFE. No matter how fierce the symptoms, no matter what the picture, no matter how long you have suffered keep your eyes, your heart, and your hope on the Path of LIFE before you. Though you may have to deal with it on some level, never become mesmerized by it. Never stare at it long enough for it to become a part of the deep-down-inside, real you."
– Michele O'Donnell from her book *Of Monkeys and Dragons: The Freedom from the Tyranny of Disease*

Especially early on in my journey, I experienced periods of time of being overtaken by this victim mentality, which I think many people with chronic illness do. And that's okay, but know that staying in this low vibrational state of fear, anger, and victimhood will not get you well. I'm actually really fortunate that my husband did an incredible job of not letting me get stuck in my "stuff" and I used many a note card pinned to walls to help keep my mindset in a positive place. It's super helpful to have friends or people in your life that can look beyond the symptoms and help you remember the Truth of who you are and hold your vision of health and happiness for you when you forget. We will talk more about creating a vision in the next chapter and the importance of having a support team later in this book.

The Hustler

While I may have had moments of victimhood, I was a bona fide grade-A hustler extraordinaire. Being the Type A, dedicated athlete that I was my whole life, I poured all my time, tenacity, and a lot of money into researching and reading, seeking out healers, and trying thousands of supplements and treatments in hopes that they would "fix" me. I thought if I could just find that one miracle supplement or pill, then I would be well. I thought if I worked hard enough at this healing thing, that I would be healed. While I did learn many things, and experienced some improvement in my symptoms, the desperate and frenetic way in which I was living was actually undermining my healing efforts.

You may also identify with this hustler mindset. This way of living and attempting to deal with your current life situation is stressful, exhausting, and only perpetuates your current reality of not feeling well. Stress depletes your immune system and sabotages your ability to heal. The hustler gives her power away by being so busy and so focused on fixing, fighting, forcing, and trying to figure it all out that she does not listen to her own heart and inner guidance to make decisions and has a hard time trusting in her body's ability to heal. She believes that healing will only happen by extreme effort, finding the right doctor, pill, or treatment, and doing all the right things.

Both the victim and the hustler give their power away by living, thinking, and acting in such a way that drains them of the vital life-force energy that is essential for healing. Blaming others or situations outside yourself or relying solely on other people or modalities to heal you may be blocking your ability to heal and keeping you from being able to access the answers you are seeking. Interestingly enough, the answers that you seek are always already inside of you and can be accessed by learning to trust yourself and slow down long enough to listen.

Take Responsibility for Your Life

You are responsible for your life. What is happening in your external reality or life circumstances is often a reflection of what's taking place within your mind. When something difficult happens to us we are often quick to blame other people or events or things, versus looking at ourselves more deeply. When we blame others, we feel justified or righteous and slip easily into that victim mindset. When we do this, we give our power away and lose the ability to learn from our experience or create a different outcome or possibility by staying stuck in the blame game and in depleting emotional states such as resentment and fear. Staying stuck here perpetuates more of the same in your life experience. Falling into victim mode can be seductive at times and sneak up on us if we aren't careful.

You, my sister, are the co-captain of *your* ship and the co-creator of *your* life. You will learn in the chapters to come that you are a creative being (whether you realize it or not), along with God, creating your life through your beliefs, thoughts, words, feelings, and actions. Therefore, you must learn to take responsibility for what's currently happening in your life in order to create a new possibility. Begin to ask your heart these important questions: *What's my part in this perceived predicament that I am in? What am I to learn here? In what ways of believing, thinking, feeling, and living have I participated in that are not in alignment with the Truth of who I am?* This is where the heart work comes in and where we take responsibility for removing the things in our life that keep us from healing and remembering who we really are.

On the other hand, it's also important to realize that we will never fully know all the reasons why things happen the way they do in our lives and in the world at large. For example, I know in my heart of hearts that part of my purpose on this planet is to help other women to heal and remember who they are. I wouldn't be doing this work if I had not gone through what I have gone through. We must not turn this understanding of our co-creative power around and blame and berate ourselves for experiencing sickness in our bodies. Time and energy spent thinking these things will not do you any good. Instead, have compassion for yourself and know that you are always doing the best you can with the information and level of awareness that you currently have (and so is everyone else). Let this understanding of your creative ability empower you to know that you have the power within to heal and alter the course of your life toward more wholeness, peace, love, fulfillment, and well-being.

The Power to Choose – Disease as a Divine Opportunity

Another way of looking at responsibility has to do with your response-ability, or your ability to respond to the situations and circumstances of your life. You actually have the power to *choose* how you will respond to this illness or the unwanted symptoms you are facing! We may not be able to fully control the events or circumstances of our lives, but we all have the power to choose our attitudes and how we will respond – whether we realize it or not.

One of my favorite quotes of all time, by Holocaust survivor, author, psychiatrist and neurologist Viktor Frankl, illustrates this beautifully:

> *"Between stimulus and response there is a space. In that space is the power to choose your response. And in that response, lies your growth and freedom."*

Take a moment to let this sink in. So many of us forget or don't realize we have a choice in how we will respond in any given moment. We often unconsciously react out of fear or anger instead of realizing we can consciously choose our responses. The outcome and trajectory of our lives is often significantly different depending on how we choose to respond.

Let me ask you this:

Will this disease be your divine opportunity – a catalyst for growth, freedom, love, peace, joy, wholeness, and reconnecting to the Truth of who you are– or will you live in constant fear and suffering, imprisoned by this illness, and let it take you over and ruin your life?

It is your choice. You may not feel like you have a choice, but you do. I've let disease keep me locked in chains, suffering and imprisoned for years. I let too many years slip by not fully awake or alive. As I've mentioned, cancer forced me to face the possibility of death head-on, took me right up against the edge of who I thought I was, and exposed many fears that bubbled to the surface to be healed. I faced my fear of dying and in doing so, I realized that I was afraid to die mostly because I hadn't ever fully lived. The realization was equally tragic and liberating. It was quite a profound and sobering moment for me. Perhaps you can relate. So, what's the antidote to not fully living? Get busy living fully *now*! And that is what I chose. I chose to see this presence of disease in my life as my opportunity to get busy fully living and loving with my whole heart. It was this shift that led to profound healing and to a level of richness and depth of life experience that I didn't know was possible. This book provides a framework for you to do the same, but ultimately it all begins with your choice of how you will respond to what is happening right now in your life.

Accepting What Is

When a challenging experience like disease is occurring in your life experience, one of the best, most helpful and powerful (and counterintuitive and often difficult at first) ways to choose to respond is to accept it. Before you get all riled up, hear me out. I'm not saying agree with what's happening, or do nothing about it, be happy about it, or throw a party about it. I am just suggesting that you choose to accept it. Here's why. So often when something we don't particularly want shows up in our lives we resist the heck out of it, wish it wasn't so, lament, try to figure out why this happened to us, waste a ton of energy in the process, and suffer tremendously. What you resist persists. Acceptance is about letting go of the resistance to what *is* and creates an opening and allowance for new possibility to arrive on the scene. Acceptance is the foundation for healing.

Have you ever lost something important, started freaking out and frantically looking for it for hours and then finally (after much searching) stopped and accepted that you may never find it again? You decide to relax. You make a cup of tea, kick your feet up on the couch, physically and emotionally exhausted after scavenging your home like a wild woman, and then bam ... you remember exactly where you left it. "Oh yes, that's right, I put it in my sock drawer for safekeeping!" You set your tea down, go to the sock drawer, and there it is! Once you let go and accepted that you may not find it, the frenzy and stress dissolved. Now in a calmer state, you were able to think more clearly and you remembered and found what you were looking for.

The energy of resistance keeps you stuck and closes off your heart and mind from receiving gifts of insight and guidance. Acceptance allows for "peace that passes all understanding" in the midst of the most challenging situations. In this place of peace, you will be much better able to listen to your heart, make decisions for your highest and best good, and is a state much more conducive to healing than the frantic state of fear and resistance.

I remember shortly after I found the lump in my breast there was a complete exasperation and utter deflation. I had been spinning my wheels (a hustler through and through) for so many years desperately trying to heal myself. To end up with cancer was a slap in the face, or at least that's how I felt – okay, more like a two by four to the head, if I'm being honest. I resisted it at first. Why me? I was angry, sad, and afraid. I desperately wanted it all to go away. I knew I couldn't stay in this place of resistance. It was too dark, too confusing, and too scary. I realized I needed to accept what was happening and surrender. I had nothing left to do but throw my hands in the air and say, "Here, God, you take this. I've got nothing left." I admit, it wasn't easy at first to accept what was happening. It was when I finally surrendered to the fact that I knew nothing, that I was prompted to go within and ask, *"What am I missing?" "What am I to learn here?"* I finally began to hear the inner promptings of my heart. God began to teach me what I had been missing. The experience of cancer became a time of much learning and growing and a catalyst for the awakening of my authentic self. It can be for you too.

How Will You Respond?

Taking responsibility for your health and this one life that you have allows you to reclaim your power, puts you in the driver's seat of your life, and prompts you to begin to look within for the answers and guidance that will best serve you. You may not always be able to control what happens in your life, but you can always control how you choose to respond. I invite you right now to think about how you will respond to your current life situation. Perhaps all you can really grasp is the prison bars you are peering out from in your current circumstance. I completely understand how that feels.

When the presence of disease and unpleasant symptoms pops up in your life it's common to get stuck in fear, resist it, and want it to go away. However, once you choose acceptance you create an opening for new possibilities and will experience less suffering, more peace, and better insight and ability to make quality decisions. Choose to accept, trust, and let go, and above all else choose love. Love is the energy in which healing takes place. I'm inviting you to begin to open to the possibility that this circumstance and these struggles can be your greatest strength and a pathway to transformation and a richer, more fulfilling life.

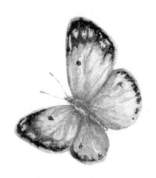

Chapter 4:

Essential #2 –
Create a Vision: Harness Your
Power to Heal

"You are the master creator of your reality.
It is your imagination that holds the key.
Unlock your treasure chest and open your heart.
Pour out all your love and live the part.
All your dreams are waiting for you.
Love yourself and follow through."
– Hafiz

A couple of years ago, not too long after my mastectomy, Chad and I renewed our vows in a sweet and intimate ceremony by the lake with our closest friends. At the ceremony, Fran handed me a very special card. It meant so much to me that she was there because she had been such a support and profound teacher for me throughout my healing journey. Inside the card she inscribed this quote by Hafiz. When I read it, I felt like I had just received a magical secret from the Universe and it resonated as Truth deep within my heart. I cut it out and taped the quote to the inside of my journal and I began reading it every morning. These new ideas of being "a master creator of your reality," the power of imagination, and the importance of opening and living from my heart and loving myself were coming into my world, not just in this Hafiz quote, but from all directions, in many different ways and from several different sources and teachers. It had my attention and I felt that I was beginning to tap into essential and Universal truths of healing and happiness – and that all I needed to do was follow the bread crumbs.

As I started walk this path of healing and wholeness, I began to open my heart and look deeper inside myself for the answers. I started to slowly realize significant and subtle ways I was sabotaging my health by holding tightly to limiting beliefs and negative and repetitive thoughts, staying stuck in fear and survival mode, as well as suppressing negative emotions and speaking words that weren't aligned with Truth and Love – all of which have creative power. Ultimately, the bread crumbs were showing me that I had a choice in the matter of my life and that I could harness the power of my imagination, beliefs, thoughts, words, and feelings by aligning them consistently with Love and my vision of vibrant health. As I did this, I began to notice subtle and the more powerful shifts inside me and experience healing in my body and life. I felt less and less at the mercy of disease and a victim of my circumstances. I began to imagine, to create a vision for my life, to trust in my power to heal, and to live in place of possibility versus being afraid all the time. These things became vitally important in helping me to shift my mindset and to begin to heal my life.

You, my love, are the co-creator of your life and the architect of your reality. Yes, your imagination holds the key and so do your thoughts, beliefs, words, and feelings – all of which are energy and have creative power that culminates to make up your life experiences – including your experience of health or disease. Understanding this becomes an essential part of your healing path so that you can realize ways in which you may be sabotaging your own healing and begin to believe, think, feel, and speak in alignment with your wholeness and that which your heart desires to experience.

We Are All Energy

You and the entire Universe are made of energy. Every person, every thing, every animal, every tree, every rock, every planet, every galaxy, is all made of the same fundamental substance – energy. Thanks to quantum physics we now know that the atoms that make up matter are actually made of 99.9999999% energy and .00001% solid stuff. Essentially, all physical things, like your body or the chair you are sitting in is actually more energy or no-thing than it is an actual thing or solid substance. Our human bodies are essentially "organized patterns of energy and information" and we are each connected to this quantum field of invisible intelligence.[4] This intelligent matrix is able to organize itself into subatomic particles, to atoms, to molecules, and to matter, and ultimately creates you, me, and all the things in the Universe.

The "observer effect" phenomenon described by quantum physicists shows the power we have to alter our reality. Essentially, the "observer effect" describes how the act of observing subatomic particles, such as an electron, changes its behavior. Scientists found that the subatomic particles that make up matter and all things (including you and me) could be either a particle or a wave depending on the person observing it. In other words, our attention or just by looking at these quantum particles changes them! We also know that the physical body down to our DNA responds to our own thinking and feeling, which we will talk more about in a moment.

A few hundred years ago, we used to believe and operate from the Newtonian physics model, which led us to an understanding that matter was made of solid particles and energy was a separate force apart from matter. This understanding meant that we didn't have much control or ability to alter our environment. Quantum physics, however, shows us that this understanding is no longer accurate. We know now that matter is made mostly of empty space and energy and that we, as the observers of our own reality, can powerfully influence matter, our environment, our bodies and life experience. This extraordinary shift in our understanding and belief moves us from being passive observers of our lives to being able to alter our life experiences, which has amazing implications for healing and manifesting our dreams. I find that Dr. Dispenza's book, *Breaking the Habit of Being Yourself: How to Lose Your Mind and Create a New One* is a fantastic introduction to these concepts, if you want to learn more.

We tend to see our lives and what is possible for ourselves from a very narrow viewpoint. Our beliefs and buying into what our culture and those around us think about "the way things are" often keeps us extremely limited in our thinking and holds us back in many ways. A great teacher of mine always reminded me that 99.99% of what is possible in my life is off my radar screen. Just knowing that we live in a field of pure potential and possibility and that we can influence our reality and our bodies with our thoughts and feelings completely changes everything and invites us all into a life of co-creation with the Infinite and being able to harness our power to heal. To do this, we must move from being stuck in fear or survival mode to living and operating more often from a place of possibility, love, and co-creation. The good news is that we have choice in the matter!

Fear vs. Love

So many people on the planet, especially those dealing with chronic illness or health challenges, are living in survival mode. We are just trying to make it through the day feeling nowhere close to our best, running ragged, and hoping to dodge any obstacles that may come our way. In survival mode, we are typically operating from this place of *fear*, lack, and stress and if we stay stuck here, we are going to have a hard time healing.

Gerald Jampolsky, author of *Love is Letting Go of Fear*, talks about letting go of fear as an essential part of healing and I couldn't agree more. It is the chronic and perpetual fear and all its derivations, such as shame, guilt and resentment, that creates disorder in our bodies, hijacks the mind, and robs us of our joy and peace. Fear operates at a low vibrational frequency (vibrational frequency being how energy is measured) which can negatively impact the body when experienced chronically. Love on the other hand is a high vibrational frequency; it raises the vibration of the body, and is where the healing happens. The good news is that at any given moment we can choose love instead of fear. *A Course in Miracles* teaches that love is what we are born with and fear is what we have learned. Healing involves a letting go of the fear and returning to who we are as Love.

Stress

In our modern era it seems like survival mode, exhaustion, and stress is the status quo, which I believe is a key reason why we have so many chronically ill people on the planet. We know that chronic stress is intimately related to disease and poor health. The American Medical Association has noted that stress is the basic cause of more than 60% of all human illness and disease *and* has been linked to most chronic disease conditions, including the six leading causes of death: heart disease, cancer, lung ailments, accidents, cirrhosis of the liver, and suicide.[5] Experiencing chronic stress has also been known to worsen the severity and prognosis of those dealing with chronic illness.

We all experience potential stressors in our lives, but the key is learning to manage it in order to avoid the negative effects on the mind and body. Stress is often thought of as something that happens to us, but it actually has more to do with how we perceive, think, and especially *feel* about the situations and events in our lives. We are designed to appropriately deal with *acute* stress in order to survive. This is a helpful and normal part of life. The hard-wired stress response that occurs in our bodies when we perceive something as stressful and potentially harmful is commonly referred to as the "fight or flight" response and is designed to help us flee, fight, and fix in order to survive potential hazardous threats. This stress response has always been an essential part of keeping us safe and is designed to keep us out of harm and to help us survive.

Here's what happens to your body when it goes into "fight or flight": certain hormones, such as adrenaline and cortisol, are released from your adrenal glands to prepare you for action. Your sympathetic nervous system kicks on, causing your respiratory and heart rates to increase, your pupils to dilate and your sight to sharpen, your awareness to intensify, and your blood to be shunted to your brain and extremities to prepare you physically and mentally to best fight or flee the situation. This mechanism is designed to be an acute response to help you run from a saber-tooth tiger or jump in to save a drowning child. It's a very important response to help you survive and keep you and your loved ones safe and is meant for acute and rare situations. However, in modern times we are constantly and chronically activating this "fight or flight" response, which is damaging to our bodies. Why does this happen, you might be asking? Because the body doesn't know the difference between being chased by a saber-tooth tiger or constantly and continuously worrying and thinking about being chased by one.

In modern day living we aren't dealing with the threat of being chased by saber-tooth tigers, but we are constantly worrying, fearing, and fretting about what happened in the past or what might happen in the future. The body responds to what we hold in our minds and responds with the same "fight or flight" response whether the threat is real or imagined. The majority of the thoughts we think are negative and repetitive, which are typically coupled with negative and depleting feelings such as fear, and anxiety, which kick on the "fight or flight" stress response. We incessantly worry we won't get the job, that our kids will get in with the wrong crowd, that our husband is cheating, that we will blow the interview, that we won't be able to pay the bills, that we may never find our purpose or be fulfilled, that we might get sick or get cancer, or, if we have cancer, we might not get well, or we might die. And the cycle goes on and on. Being in this chronically stressed state is known to cause detrimental effects on the body including inflammation, premature aging, weakening of the immune system, anxiety, depression, weight gain, blood sugar dysregulation, hormone imbalances, muscle loss, sleep disturbances, impaired cognition and memory, headaches, and digestive issues.

When we are stuck in fear, stress, and in survival mode, not only does it wreak havoc on the body, it leads to disease and prevents us from healing. Living and leading from our heads versus our hearts like we talked about in the last chapter often keeps us in survival mode and fear. Spending most of our lives in this state sabotages our health and keeps us from living the lives we desire, make decisions for our highest good, and keeps us stuck, confused, and overwhelmed.

Fear and the Deer

One evening during my mastectomy recovery, Chad and I were returning home from an evening stroll. We were walking hand in hand in the parking lot right outside the condo where we were staying and I saw something strange up ahead. We stopped about twenty yards in front of the tennis court. The tennis court was enclosed by an extremely tall chain link fence, which had two doors swung open, one at each diagonal of the rectangular court. Inside of the tennis court was a deer. I nudged Chad and we both stopped to watch. She must've meandered through one of the open doors and obviously found herself in a very peculiar place. She was clearly scared and started darting around, unsure of what to do. And then it happened. She ran full speed from one side of the tennis court to the other and attempted to jump over the fence. Smack! Her body crashed into the chain-link fence and she fell to the ground with a thud that made me cry out. Oh no! I looked at Chad. "Why did she do that?" I said.

"She doesn't see the open doors. She's too afraid," he said.

The deer lay there for a minute, stunned. But then she slowly got up and shook herself off. Then to our amazement and horror, she reared up and did it again in a different direction. Smack! And then … thud. She was bleeding this time. I started crying. I ran inside the condo to get some carrots, hoping that if I put them by the open exit she would see it. Nope. She was in such a state of stress and terror that my presence only made her more skittish. We backed away and I tried to call for help, but no animal clinics would come to rescue an adult deer, only fawns.

She proceeded to run and jump into the fence and fall to the ground three more times until she could no longer get up. We watched, tears flowing down my face, as she tried to stand up using her front legs, but she couldn't get up because her back legs were broken. Her mouth was bloodied. She attempted to scoot, but she barely moved. It was painful to watch, but we didn't want to leave her. All she had to do was walk through the open doors! There wasn't just one door, but there were two, for heaven's sake. *C'mon sweetheart, why couldn't you have just walked through the same way that you came in?* I thought. It was so simple. *How come she didn't realize this?* I got this sense that I was supposed to learn something here. I was beginning to become accustomed to finding teachers and messages in all different shapes, sizes, and forms in my life. *God, why did I see this? What am I to learn?* And this is what came to me:

"*There are always openings, my love,*" I heard. "*You're just too stuck in your head to notice them. I always provide a way.*"

I started to sob. Oh, how many times had I been that deer! I've spent so much of my life in a state of chronic stress and fear. And in my frenzied state I would charge forward and end up running into walls, bloodying and bruising myself, when the whole time if I would've stopped, slowed down, asked for guidance, and listened to my heart, I would have seen the wide-open door to my freedom. I thanked God for the insight and honored the deer for teaching me such a valuable lesson.

Can you relate to the deer? How often do you find yourself going through life at a frenzied pace looking for a way out and feeling bloodied and bruised? You don't have to be the deer anymore. The way out of fear, overwhelm, suffering, and the stranglehold of disease is through the heart. That's where the opening always resides. The answers or the openings are always there – you have to learn to slow down and listen within. The answers you are seeking are already inside you. I don't have all the answers when it comes to your life and your challenges, but you do. I'm only providing a roadmap back to your own heart. We must move away from staying stuck in the past and future in our minds, allowing the head to run the show, attaching to the repetitive fearful and negative thoughts and continually experiencing the same depleting and anxious emotions. Chronic and continuous negative thoughts and emotions keep us in a perpetual "fight or flight" or stressful states and make us sick. But the good news is that when we slow the breath and think and feel greater than our current experience, we can snap out of the "fight or flight" fearful state and move to the "rest, repair, and rejuvenate" state that is so essential to healing. It is the syncing of our minds with our hearts, returning to love and the present moment, trusting in our heart, asking for guidance, and feeling the renewing emotions of the heart (love, gratitude, care, and compassion) that allows us to tap into our power to heal, make the best decisions for our lives, access our intuition, and consciously create a life that we truly love.

We Are Creative Beings

We are actually always creating, whether we realize it or not. When we are stuck in fear and survival mode we continue to create more of the same and wonder why we cannot break through to the experiences we deeply desire in life. Some of us live our whole lives like the deer trying to escape the tennis court, but we don't have to anymore. When we are able to access our hearts and return to a state of harmony we see that the door was open the whole time and walk through it with ease.

Thanks to quantum physics, we can now step into the knowing of ourselves as conscious co-creators of our reality and begin tapping into this power to heal and manifest the desires of our hearts. How can we learn to create more health, well-being, and love in our lives? What do you want to experience in this life? How do you want to feel? How do you want to be different? Let these thoughts begin to percolate in your consciousness.

I know for me and many women that are struggling with the pain, fear, doubt, and overwhelm that often accompanies chronic disease that it is easy to get stuck in the negative vortex of it all. These questions that I have posed may feel like a frivolous use of your energy and a waste of time.

But, stick with me – these very questions can be the portal to improving your health and your life.

I know that sometimes it may feel like you are barely able to make it through the day and handle all the challenges life appears to be throwing at you, on top of feeling sick. You may be stuck in survival mode, just hoping to get through the day without things getting worse. Of course, you want to feel vibrant and amazing, vacation on the beautiful beaches of Bali and dance the tango with a hot Latin lover, but you stopped dreaming because the dream is in such stark contrast to your current reality that it hurts too much to indulge in such thoughts. However, it is these dreams and your imagination that can help pull you out of the quicksand and build the bridge to a different life starring a healthier, happier you.

I know I wouldn't be where I am now without Chad. There were so many times and instances in the past decade where he showed up powerfully with his loving presence, wisdom, and unconditional love. Knowing what I know now about quantum physics and the power of thoughts and feelings to create, there is one particular thing he said to me that probably saved my life. Remember back when I was sick in bed, on disability, covered in rashes, and wanted to die? I couldn't do much but lay there covered in ice packs. I remember Chad coming into the room and lying next to me. I can't remember what we were talking about, but he asked me what my dream was. He asked me to describe a particular experience that I dreamed of having. I was annoyed at first. "I don't know," I told him. "C'mon, just do it," he said. "If you could go anywhere, do anything and feel what you most want to feel … what would that look like?" I rolled my eyes and then obliged and closed my eyes to contemplate.

To my surprise, my imagination took me to a gorgeous beach with the waves crashing on the shore and the sun brightly shining. I was in a colorful bikini, with clear, healthy tan skin, a strong body and walking hand in hand with Chad. We were smiling, talking, and laughing. I felt light and free. We decided to work out on the beach together doing squats, planks, and crawling in the sand (working out was something we used to do together, but I was no longer able to). When we were finished and had worked up a sweat, he scooped me up and ran into the surf up to his waist. I squealed with delight and laughed as we got soaked by the waves. He put me down and I clasped my hands around the back of his neck and kissed him. We walked hand in hand back down the beach looking at all the beautiful flowers, the birds, and the sunset. I felt happy, healthy, strong, free, and filled with love and appreciation for the moment. I smiled and opened my eyes and proceeded to tell Chad about everything I saw. Just by imagining my dream and feeling the feelings of my wish fulfilled created a change in me. I felt more relaxed and I even smiled. He smiled and assured me that my dream would come true one day.

From that day on, I imagined this scenario every single day. I felt what it would feel like to have clear skin again, to be healthy, and to be free and full of energy. It never failed to make me smile and feel better. Years later this scenario played out in real life on the beautiful beaches of Costa Rica. I was overwhelmed with joy as Chad and I walked hand in hand down the beach. I couldn't believe that this vision I'd been rehearsing in my mind and feeling world was playing out in real time. I savored the sand under my feet, the sea breeze, and the sun bronzing my clear, rash-free skin. I was beyond grateful. I didn't know it then, but I was beginning to learn how to activate the power of my imagination to heal and co-create my life.

Thoughts + Feelings – It's Where the Magic Is

Our thoughts have creative power, but not nearly as strong as our thoughts combined with our feelings. Dr. Joe Dispenza describes this "thinking and feeling loop" in which thinking and feeling reinforce each other. For example, thinking about your coworker who pissed you off earlier today in your business meeting creates chemicals in your body that make you have feelings of anger – sensations of heat in your face and perhaps a contracted sensation in your chest. The feelings in the body further perpetuate the thinking and you begin to think of other times that this particular coworker pissed you off. This unified thought + feeling creates a "state of being" that radically affects your life experience.[6] Often we get stuck in a rut, so to speak, and memorize these states of being – let's say, "I am a victim" or "I'm a fearful person" or "a sad person," – then it gets hard-wired and conditioned in our mind and body and becomes a habit or automatic program. Unfortunately, the majority of the time these automatic programs that we have memorized are running the show and we don't even realize it.

You may decide you want to "be happy," instead of sad. You know that being happy and more at ease will help you heal, but the body has been programmed for years to produce those "sad" chemicals that coincide with those sad thoughts. Just thinking "happy thoughts" won't be enough. You've got to combine the happy thoughts with the new feelings you wish to experience. It's about thinking and feeling beyond what is currently happening in your reality. It's thinking, feeling, and living as if your dream has already happened that allows the creative and healing juices to flow!

Here's an incredible example of how intentional thought + heart-based positive feelings can powerfully alter our bodies – even our DNA! There was a study conducted through the HeartMath Institute that demonstrated that DNA strands could be influenced by heart-focused intention. Participants held 3 test tubes of DNA in their hands and were instructed to get into a state of heart coherence and set an intention to simultaneously unwind two out of three of the DNA samples and leave the third one unchanged. Heart coherence is a state of physical, mental, and emotional harmony that is achieved using a HeartMath technique that consists of heart-focused breathing and intentional positive emotions (more on how to do this in Chapter 6). Those individuals that were able to get into that place of high coherence were able to unwind the DNA strands as instructed with the power of their thinking and feeling! How amazing is that?! Those that exhibited low coherence were not effective at altering the DNA. The positive emotions were key! If we have the power to unwind DNA strands that contain our genetic blueprint, think about the possibilities of being able to heal our bodies through our intentional thoughts and emotions![7]

Creating a Vision and Intention

In *Breaking the Habit of Being Yourself: How to Lose Your Mind and Create a New One*, Dr. Dispenza explains, "when you've 'experienced' an event numerous times by mentally rehearsing every aspect of it in your mind, you feel what that event would feel like, before it unfolds. Then as you change circuitry in your brain by thinking in new ways, and you embrace the emotions of an event ahead of its physical manifestation, it's possible that you can change your body genetically."

When we create a vision for our health and life of what we want to experience and we repeatedly think and visualize it, and then combine that with the feeling of that wish fulfilled, we begin to rewire those hard-wired programs and the body begins to respond as if it's already happening. The key is repetition and deep feeling. Remember, the body doesn't know the difference between being chased by a saber-tooth tiger or just thinking and worrying about it. The stress response occurs either way. And when we repeatedly envision our new desired reality with deep feeling, we activate positive, healing chemicals in the body and begin to influence the quantum field and Divine Intelligence to consciously co-create a life or experience that we desire. It is all about aligning our thoughts and feelings with our wish fulfilled and thinking and feeling greater than our current circumstances. This is where the magic is!

When you are dealing with chronic illness, it's so easy to slip into the abyss of your endless and ongoing problems. I know it can be hard to get out of, but as you've learned, you have a choice and you can activate your power to create something different. One of my mentors once told me, "It's better to be pulled by your vision than pushed by your problems." In order to harness our power to heal and consciously create a life we love, we *must* be pulled by our vision and begin to live from our wish fulfilled. Creating a vision and re-visiting that vision and daily (repetition) and aligning your thoughts, words, and feelings with this vision is perhaps one of the most important tools you can implement to help you heal and create an extraordinary life. And, guess what? It's absolutely free. I will show you how.

Whole-Hearted Vision Book

I recommend creating what I like to call a Whole-Hearted Vision Book, which will help you to revisit your health and life visions on a daily basis. This binder will contain your health and life visions in visual format.

To make one you will need the following: a three-ring binder, white paper or construction paper, a three-hole punch, a pen or markers, scissors, a glue stick, and old magazines and/or a computer to print out pictures.

Prep-Work: Journaling

But, before you actually create anything, grab a pen and paper and go to a quiet comfortable spot, perhaps a beautiful place that makes you feel happy, relaxed, and safe. You are going to begin to communicate with your heart. What are the desires of your heart? It's time to allow yourself to dream again. Close your eyes and let the labels, diagnoses, presence of symptoms, the pain, all that has happened in the past, the fear of the future, the thoughts of "I can't," "There's no way," "why bother" all fall away. Take a moment to connect with your breath and feel into your heart. Don't forget, you are a piece of God in action – a co-creator of your reality. You are magnificent!

Now, imagine yourself a year from now. You have won the lottery and now have in your possession one hundred million dollars! You have all the money you can possibly imagine at your disposal. What is that you want to be doing and feeling? Where will you go? Who are you with? What are you doing? What will you create? How does it feel in your body? Let the visions and the feelings come. Write them down in your notebook and hold nothing back. Dream big and then dream bigger. Give yourself full permission to dream without limitations. Do the same exact thing for five years and ten years. Write each vision down on separate pieces of paper and push the limits of your imagination.

Create Your Collage

Now once you have your written one-, five-, and ten-year visions, you get to create visual representations for each in the form of a collage. Let the creativity that you had when you were a kid come out to play and have fun! Use a standard piece of white computer paper or construction paper for your collage. You will hole punch these and put them in your binder. Take some time to cut out images of pictures from old magazines or print pictures and words out from the computer and cut them out. These pictures and words will symbolize and remind you of your written dreams and vision. Paste them on your white paper or construction paper. Be sure to use bright colors and images that make you feel good. Feel free to use more than one page per vision.

How to Use It

I recommend spending a few minutes with your Whole-Hearted Vision Book every morning as part of your morning routine. We will talk more about the power of an awesome morning practice in Chapter 12. Take your time to look over your one-, five-, and ten-year collages. Imagine experiencing these things. Activate the feelings that accompany your images or words. Remember, the feeling is key! What would it be like for these things to be made manifest? Again, I recommend doing this every morning, and you can also do this in the evening before bed or anytime you feel afraid or doubtful. It is the daily practice of this and the repetition, combined with activating your imagination, visualization, and deep feeling that makes this so powerful.

Approach this time of imagination with a spirit of gratitude, openness, and acknowledgment that we are co-creators and don't have it all figured out. We are not expecting God to do everything we say when we say it. We know that there are ways and plans bigger and grander than we could understand and we are ultimately trusting in divine perfect order and surrendering our dreams and desires of our heart to God. Remember, God knows us better than we know ourselves and always has our best interest at heart.

I have all my clients do this and it has been such a powerful tool for so many of them! One client shared with me that this was the one thing that helped her more than anything when she started worrying about her health and her future. Most women dealing with chronic illness have to overcome varying levels of fear, doubt, and overwhelm (sometimes on a daily basis) in order to heal and live lives they desire. This practice is life-changing and I love that it hardly costs a thing. But, you must have the discipline to *do* it!

I still look at my Whole-Hearted Vision Book every day and continue to update it as my dreams unfold. I have an image on my five-year vision of a book, symbolizing me writing this book you are reading now. And it just so happens that it has come to fruition in one year instead of five! It's so fun to watch your intentions unfold – sometimes in the way you visualize and sometimes so much better! Stay open and flexible!

Intention

An intention is a thought to do, create, or become something or someone. All dreams begin with an intention, like sowing a seed. Daily repetition of speaking an intention aloud is like watering the seeds to help it begin to grow. Evoking the feelings of the fulfillment of this intention is like the sunshine that is necessary for it to blossom and reach its full potential. When we create a daily intention (thought) that is representative of our dream come true and we use language that indicates it has already happened or is currently so, such as "I am vibrantly healthy," and combine it with a little water (speak it aloud with our word) and add sunshine (deep feeling) we tap further into our own power to create.

Power of the Word

Combining thought + feeling with repetition is key to reprogramming our subconscious mind and influencing the quantum field to create the desires of our heart. Adding the power of the spoken word with a daily intention is like icing on the cake.

Like emotions and thoughts, words are made of energy and vibration. Words have extraordinary power to heal or harm ourselves and others. We must take responsibility and become conscious of our language. Are we speaking words that are aligned with the desires of our hearts to be well, happy, and free? Begin watching your language and note the way you speak to yourself (aloud and inside your head) and to others. You will continually improve your health and life by upgrading your language, along with upgrading your thoughts, feelings, and beliefs, which all influence your actions.

> *"Words are singularly the most powerful force available to humanity.*
> *We can choose to use this force constructively with words of*
> *encouragement, or destructively using words of despair. Words have*
> *energy and power with the ability to help, to heal, to hinder, to*
> *hurt, to harm, to humiliate and to humble."*
> – Yehuda Berg

Have you seen the experiments performed in the late 90s and early 2000s by Masaru Emoto?[8] He conducted several experiments looking at the effect of language or intention on the crystalline structure of water. The results and the photographs are extraordinary. Emoto put water in glasses, exposed the water to various words, prayers, and music, froze it, and looked at it under a microscope. The water exposed to positive words, such as "love" or "truth," prayers, or uplifting music created stunning, orderly, complex, and beautiful shapes similar to snowflakes. However, when the water was exposed to negative phrases or words such as "you disgust me" and "evil" or heavy metal music, distorted and disorderly shapes were created. I highly recommend looking this up and seeing the pictures yourself. They are fascinating!

These experiments profoundly demonstrate the impact our words have on living things such as water. Did you know that the human body is made of approximately 60% water? Our health and well-being as individuals and collectively are most definitely altered and affected by the words we speak aloud and in our minds, but also by the words and music we are exposed to. It's important to be mindful of the music you listen to, the movies you watch, and the people that you spend time with. Surround yourself with love, beauty and life-affirming words, music, people and experiences!

Create a Ninety-Day Intention

I highly recommend creating a ninety-day intention in conjunction with your Whole-Hearted Vision book that will be part of your daily morning practice. You can type this or handwrite it. Put one copy of your finalized intention on your bathroom mirror and the other copy in your three-ring binder. To craft your intention, use language that indicates that what you desire is happening now. Use language that indicates what you want to happen, versus what you do not want to happen.

For example:
- Don't use: I am not overweight anymore.
- Use: I am healthy. I love my body and I feel good in my own skin.

What do you desire to experience? What do you desire to feel? What do you desire to have? Choose things that feel like a stretch, but don't feel so impossible that you don't believe it could ever happen. For example, for me to win an Olympic Gold medal in ice skating would be awesome, however I've only ice skated once in my life and am past the prime age of an Olympic ice-skating champion. This is not a reasonable intention for me. I don't personally believe that this could ever happen, nor do I really want to put in the energy or work to make it happen!

Here are some examples I've used in the past:
- I am vibrantly healthy with clear, smooth skin.
- I live from my heart and listen to my heart.
- I trust in my body to heal.
- I have a beautiful home that I love, that's comfortable and peaceful to be in, and is surrounded by nature.
- I have a group of dear sister friends that I connect deeply and intimately with.
- I have a co-empowered, passionate, and fun relationship with my husband.

Start each day by stating your intention *out loud* in the mirror. I do this after I brush my teeth in the morning. It's a good idea to ground yourself by taking a few deep breaths in and out of your heart. Look at yourself in the mirror and say your intention aloud three times. Don't forget to *feel* the feelings of what it will feel like to be vibrantly healthy or have that home surrounded by nature! Invoke a feeling of gratitude that what you desire has already happened. Stick with the same intention for ninety days. After ninety days, update your intention, but not before. You may realize that some things have come to fruition and you don't need to keep them any longer. Feel free to add new intentions at this time.

Harness Your Power to Heal

It is in harnessing the power of your thoughts, words, feelings, and beliefs, and imagining greater than your current reality that you can manifest and create the desires of your heart and activate your healing potential. Before something has become a reality it was born in thought and vision first. That is why creating a vision and intention for your health and life is absolutely essential!

Before anyone ever walked on the moon, someone thought it might be possible and began to cultivate that dream into reality. Martin Luther King Jr. had a dream that brothers and sisters of different races and skin colors would sit down at the same table and live as equals during a time when it was hard to believe that could ever happen. His belief, his passion, and his vision is what created the momentum for law to change and for people to begin to change the way they believed about segregation and racism. There are multitudes of men and women who have healed their bodies and lives from the most catastrophic illness and circumstances. They did because they believed they could and so can you!

This is your time to dream and create a vision for your health and life. It's time to stop waiting until "one day" when you are healed and begin to heal now by imagining beyond your current life situation to one in which you are well and whole. Trust in your innate power to heal and tap into your power to co-create that which you deeply desire inside your heart.

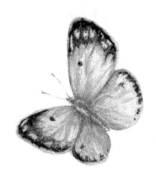

Chapter 5:

Essential #3 –
Thoughts and Beliefs

"You have the power to heal yourself, and you need to know that. We think so often that we are helpless, but we're not. We always have the power of our minds. Claim and consciously use your power."
– Louise Hay

In the last chapter, we talked about how aligning your thoughts, words, and feelings with your vision of your wish fulfilled is one of the most powerful things you can do when it comes to healing and creating a life you love. In this chapter, we will dive a little deeper into how thoughts as well as beliefs play a powerful role in the quality of your life experience and your ability to heal.

Thoughts

By now you are likely beginning to realize the inherent power of your thoughts to create on the canvas that is your life. When it comes to experiencing sickness, we are so quick to blame the body for breaking down and treating the sickness on the level of body only, that we fail to look at what is going on in our thinking and feeling worlds. It's often said that the contents of our lives are a reflection of what we hold in thought. It's essential as you navigate your healing journey that you begin to become aware of the thoughts you are thinking and empower yourself to choose those thoughts you wish to experience.

The brain is an extraordinarily powerful tool that helps you get around in this world. And what does it do best? It thinks. A lot. Often so much so that it drives us bonkers! Can you relate? The mind thinks compulsively without stopping. It is estimated that we think somewhere in the ballpark of 60,000 thoughts per day. Unfortunately, it just so happens that most of these thoughts are repetitive, negative, and not very constructive. This voice in your head is often called the "ego mind" and is dominated by fear. Its goal is safety, security and is always on high alert. It's a helpful and necessary tool, however when you let it take over and attach and identify with those negative and repetitive thoughts, you reinforce the depleting feelings that accompany those thoughts such as anxiety, worry, and fear. You end up getting stuck in that "fight or flight" stress response and ultimately create suffering, unhappiness, and disharmony in your mind and body.

But guess what? Good news! *You* are actually not your thoughts! *You* are not the voice in your head. You can take a step back as the observer of your mind and choose those thoughts that you wish to experience. Consider your highest Self as the gardener of your mind. Don't let the weeds and pests (negative thoughts) multiply and take over! Only hold on to those thoughts you wish to experience. How, you may ask? Realizing you aren't your thoughts is a powerful first step! Next, you have to practice becoming aware of your thoughts. You can't completely stop your mind from thinking negative thoughts. It's inevitable that the pests and weeds will pop up – that's okay, just don't let them set up shop.

There are tools and strategies, like meditation and practicing present moment awareness, that can help you slow down the racing thoughts and create more spaciousness for you to notice your thoughts easier. As you become more aware of the thoughts in your head, you become better at being able to choose those thoughts that are affirming, supportive, healing and uplifting and let the others pass on by. And as we discussed last chapter, thoughts and feelings are intimately connected. Consciously activating a positive heart-based emotion, like gratitude or love, can be extremely helpful in positively influencing your thoughts.

Three Parts of the Mind

There are three basic parts of the mind. The superconscious mind is the aspect of the mind that is connected with the Mind of God, or One Mind and is often called your Higher Self. The conscious mind is the part of the mind that is conscious of what is going on right now and what we are paying attention to in this moment. It's the part that is taking in information, analyzing it, and processing it in real time and only accounts for 5% or less of the cognitive activity of the day. The subconscious mind is the part of the mind that is beneath our conscious awareness, and is the one actually running the show 95% of the time!

The subconscious mind contains a record of all of the past experiences of your life. It stores all the events, situations, all the knowledge you've accumulated, the most incredible moments or challenging moments of your life, all the traumas, all the joys, and everything in between (especially information from that highly impressionable time before the age of seven when you were soaking up information like a sponge without a filter).[9] Essentially, it stores all your feelings, thoughts, memories, and beliefs about everything that has ever happened.

The subconscious mind is much bigger and faster than the conscious mind and takes care of all the automatic responses during the day using everything it has learned. Although you don't actually remember everything you've experienced, it's stored in that subconscious mind of yours and the majority of what happens in your life is influenced by it. Most of your decisions, actions, feelings and behaviors on a daily basis are directed by what is held outside of your conscious awareness. Unfortunately, often much of what is stored in the subconscious mind is negative, limiting, and disempowering and therefore we have the tendency to recreate these negative experiences in our lives.

It is through becoming aware of limiting thoughts, feelings, and beliefs and learning to think and feel greater than your circumstances, and rewriting these faulty, negative programs, that you can experience something different and new. This has powerful implications for those that are sick of being sick. You may have thought, *Why do I keep struggling with my health?* Addressing your thinking and feeling worlds and becoming aware of and releasing negative thoughts and beliefs is an important piece of the puzzle.

It's helpful to remember that many of the negative voices and messages that are playing like tapes in your mind are a result of things that happened in the past or messages that you previously picked up on. Much of this garbage is categorically untrue. However, if you don't realize you are not your thoughts and cultivate awareness of your thoughts, these voices become so loud that you can't help but begin to believe them. It's these voices that say, "You're stupid," "You're never going to heal," "You don't deserve to be well," "You're never going to be enough," or "You're ugly" that are most definitely not true. You must be diligent and not allow those thoughts to take over. Don't believe them, my dear one! These are lies and they will hold you back from healing. I find it helpful to replace these thoughts with the exact opposite. For example, "you're stupid" becomes "you're brilliant."

The Truth of you is that you are a magnificent, beautiful, unique expression of the Divine. Don't let those voices derail you from remembering who and what you are. Remembering is the key to healing and wholeness. Be an avid and alert gardener of your mind and only allow those thoughts you wish to experience and ignore or upgrade the rest! As we discussed in the previous chapter, begin to turn your thoughts toward your vision of health and avail yourself of the power of the mind to heal.

Healing Power of the Mind

Dr. Joe Dispenza's personal story is a prime and powerful example of the power of the mind to heal. If you have never read his books, I highly recommend doing so. It's a must for anyone on a healing journey to be able to know what is possible. I will provide you with the highlights of his story here.

Dispenza was in the middle of competing in a triathlon in 1996 when he was hit by a car from behind while on his bike. He sustained very serious injuries, including compression fractures of six of his vertebrae and bone shard fragments encroaching on his spinal cord. He was in quite a bit of pain and had neurological symptoms that included numbness, tingling, and loss of lower extremity function. The doctors told him he would need a major surgery that involved the placement of two stainless steel rods along the spine in order for him to have a shot of ever walking again. The top surgeon in the area recommended he move forward with the surgery, but he knew that if he did walk again he would probably live the rest of his life with chronic pain. However, the alternative, not doing the surgery, had even greater consequences, including paralysis. Dispenza didn't like either option, but ultimately decided to forego the surgery and trust in the Divine Intelligence within himself to heal.

Because of the severity of the injury, he could not do anything but lay face down. Each day he committed to surrendering to "the greater mind that has unlimited power" and focusing his conscious attention on the healing power within him and very specifically gave instructions to his body to repair his spine. He kept all thoughts focused on his desired outcome, allowing no negative thoughts to enter. At nine and a half weeks after the accident he began walking without any surgery and by twelve weeks he had returned to training again while continuing his rehabilitation. To this day he reports rarely experiencing back pain. He went on to diligently study neuroscience and teach and inspire many about the power we all have within us to heal.[10]

Watch Your Thoughts

A good way to begin bringing awareness to your thoughts is to get a notepad and set a timer for five minutes. Write down every thought that comes up. After the five minutes, see how many of your thoughts are actually positive and useful. You will likely find that most are negative or not very helpful at all.

Another good practice is to spend three days watching your thoughts very intently. Jot down the thoughts that are the most negative and repetitive. This may give you some clues as to the thoughts you are thinking that are holding you back from being well. This exercise will allow you to become more aware of your negative thoughts and the next time these thoughts pop up, you can notice them and choose something different.

Meditation

Meditation is an incredible tool for creating more awareness about your thoughts, feelings, and beliefs and has been around for thousands and thousands of years. Meditation changed my life and is one of the practices that I believe is crucial to being well. It's a practice that I have all my clients do, even if it's only for five minutes a day.

A meditation practice doesn't have to be intimidating or overwhelming. Everyone, I mean everyone, can do it and benefit from it. Hundreds of studies show a wide range of benefits of meditation including improved immune function, improved emotional resilience, increased positive emotions, decreased anxiety and stress, pain reduction, and decreased feeling of loneliness and depression. Essentially, meditation helps you to create space around your thoughts, slow down the compulsive thinking mind and also helps you to connect with your Highest Self that is beyond your mind and feeling world. By meditating you can slow down your thinking, gain some awareness about what you are thinking and feeling, better access your intuition, and choose the thoughts and feelings you most want to experience. Powerful, right?! And these benefits even spill over into your day-to-day interactions and experiences.

I have a client, Sherri, who was amazed how just by meditating five minutes a day in the morning, she was much calmer and centered in her interactions with challenging customers and during difficult conversations with her husband. After two weeks, she noticed that she no longer got "all worked up" and said things in a harsh or reactive way. She described being able to watch her negative thought in the moment, feel the frustration, but then take a breath to calm herself and respond from a loving place. This is so huge! In the last chapter, we talked about the negative impact of stress on the physical body. Through a consistent and simple meditation practice, Sherri was able to reduce stress and ultimately felt better and happier as a result.

There are many different types and variations of meditation, but essentially it involves sitting comfortably in stillness with an erect spine, closing your eyes and bringing your attention to your breath. Begin focusing your attention on the in and out flow of your breath. When your thoughts begin to wander, bring your attention lovingly back to your breath. Continue focusing on the breath until the timer goes off. That's pretty much it! You can do this in stillness or with some relaxing music in the background. Other types of meditation involve focusing on an object like a candle or saying a mantra or short word or statement over and over again. There are also guided meditations, which can be very helpful for beginners, that involve listening to a voice guiding you throughout the meditation.

Some people describe prayer as talking to God and meditation as listening to God. I like this explanation, but it does not necessarily have to take on a spiritual or religious context. Mindfulness-based stress reduction (MBSR), created by Jon Kabat-Zinn, for example is a secular meditation and mindfulness program. It is offered by several medical centers and hospitals as a useful tool for reducing stress, pain, and improving overall health and well-being.

For me, meditation creates space in my life to remember who I am, to align with Truth every morning, and to connect with God and myself. Sometimes I get insights during meditation, sometimes tears and emotions come up that I didn't know needed to come up, and sometimes it's pretty uneventful. The overall effect for me and for many is that it helps calm my mind and emotions, helps me to be more emotionally resilient throughout the day, and helps me to start the day feeling grounded, peaceful, and uplifted. It's also been a powerful tool to help me overcome fear, doubt, overwhelm, and stress, which as you know can sabotage your healing efforts.

The power of meditation is in the consistent practice. I recommend starting with five minutes in the morning and gradually increasing your practice to twenty or thirty minutes. Meditation is one of the most powerful tools for healing and upgrading your life. If you don't currently practice meditation I highly recommend that you do!

Beliefs

"She believed she could, so she did."
– R.S. Grey, *Scoring Wilder*

My dear, do you believe that you can heal? Do you believe that you deserve to be well? Have you ever stopped to take inventory of what you believe to be true about yourself, your abilities, your limitations, God, disease, health, and the world you live in? Why? Because what you believe creates the blueprint for your life. The culmination of what you believe is the lens through which you uniquely see and interpret your reality. Your thoughts, feelings, and actions, as well as the way you live your life, stem from your beliefs. There is *enormous* power in what you believe. What you believe can be a force that supports your highest good and vision for your life and can help you heal, or it can be like a ball and chain that is holding you back and limiting you in ways you don't even realize.

My intention is not to tell you what to believe, but to invite you to explore your beliefs with an open and curious mind and compassionate heart. If you are like me, you may come to realize that your beliefs about yourself and your ability to heal are holding you back from what it is that you really desire. Identifying and transforming limiting and destructive beliefs into life-affirming beliefs may be one of the most important things you can do on your path to healing and wholeness.

What is a belief? In the book *Spontaneous Healing of Belief,* Gregg Braden defines belief as the "certainty that comes from accepting what we *think* is true in our minds, coupled with what we *feel* is true in our hearts." Beliefs are like computer programs or codes that dictate what shows up on the screen of our lives. Your inner experience of belief, your accepted thoughts + feelings, communicates with Divine Intelligence and affects your day-to-day experience. Braden states that there are several ancient spiritual texts that discuss the power of combining thought + feeling that the majority of people aren't aware of, such as texts from Gnostic and Christian traditions from over two thousand years ago and in early translations of the book of John in the Bible. These ancient texts corroborate recent science that shows that we can alter our reality by combining our thoughts with feelings. Do you remember how the participants in the HeartMath study were able to unwind strands of DNA by invoking heart-based positive emotions and intentional thought? This demonstrates how we can powerfully affect our bodies and use this information to heal! If you believe you can heal, you can!

Where do our adult beliefs come from? Surprisingly, they are mostly shaped by our childhood, whether we realize it or not. Our beliefs come from all the experiences we've ever had and are heavily shaped by how we were raised and what our parents and caregivers believed about everything from religion, to science, to history, to politics, and their cultural customs and traditions. We often create beliefs about ourselves, our lives, our limitations, and our capabilities in early childhood. As mentioned, from birth to age seven we are soaking up information like sponges, mostly from our primary caregivers and family of origin, on how to be, think, feel, and relate to the world and what to believe.[11] This includes the positive and negative stuff alike, the judgments, the criticism, the praise, the behaviors, the temperaments, habits, likes/dislikes, and biases. And quite often our parents or caregiver's beliefs and ways of being in the world were in part inherited from their parents or care-givers and so on. Essentially, most of your beliefs, whether conscious or subconscious, are beliefs you've inherited from other people! Consider this – what if these beliefs are wrong or not aligned with Truth and Love, and what if they are undermining your dreams and desires to heal and be well?

I remember when I was young, probably around the age of seven or eight, and I went to eat dinner and spend the night at a friend's house for the first time ever. We were having spaghetti and meatballs with salad and breadsticks for dinner – which was one of my favorites at the time. And as we were filling our plates and passing the dishes around the table, I began wondering where the applesauce was. I looked all over and I didn't see it. *Hmmm … that's weird*, I thought. After dinner, I asked my friend why we didn't have applesauce for dinner and she looked at me like I had three heads. "Why would we have applesauce for dinner?" she asked. I told her that my family always had applesauce on the dinner table at my house. I whole-heartedly believed that everyone spanning the globe had applesauce with dinner, because that is what we did in our household. It turns out that my dad loves eating applesauce with dinner so that's why it's always on the table! This is a cute and silly example, but there are many things that are much more significant that we believe from a young age that can both positively and negatively shape our world.

Upon entering into adulthood, we rarely look at our beliefs to see if they are actually true for us. Nor do we realize that what we believe is radically impacting the very experiences we are having in our lives – including vibrant health or disease, wealth or money problems, happi-ness or depression. If you are sick and having a hard time getting well or you are just someone wanting to live their best life possible, I highly recommend taking a look at your beliefs. It is through this contemplative process that you may find some faulty programs that are sabotaging your healing efforts and keeping you from experiencing the peace, love, abun-dance, and connection you crave.

It wasn't until my late twenties, during my TaoFlow yoga training, that I was prompted to take a look at my beliefs. My teacher gave a lecture on "cosmology," or the lens through which we see the world, as he described it, and had us contemplate why we believed the things we believed. I was shocked to realize that so many of my beliefs about life, God, religion, politics, and myself were a result of what my parents believed, the religious institutions I was brought up in, and the area of the world and country in which I lived. Did *I* actually believe those things to be true, or did I just unconsciously accept them as true? Wow. I was blown away that I had never questioned something as fundamental as what I believed about such important topics.

We get in trouble when we lack the self-awareness to check in and question our beliefs. Think about atrocities that have occurred throughout history, like the Holocaust or slavery. Most people look at those two periods of time and what happened as horrible, outrageous, and unacceptable, but many "good" people believed at the time that it was okay to treat people of other races and skin colors in such inhumane ways. These people were highly influenced by governmental and religious leaders and believed that what they were doing was "right."

Refraining from questioning our beliefs or believing something because someone or some group of people says we "should" can be dangerous. Not to mention, time after time what we once collectively believed to be true, is then proved to be untrue and obsolete. Recall how at one point we believed the earth was flat or the sun revolved around the earth, which is no longer the case. It's extremely important, not only in the realm of healing, but in living our best lives possible, that we examine our beliefs and choose ones that resonate as Truth deep in our hearts and are aligned with that which we want to experience.

Becoming Aware of Limiting Beliefs

Often our limiting beliefs hang out in the subconscious mind, the part of the mind outside of our conscious awareness, and as mentioned, were formed when we were young kiddos. These limiting beliefs do exactly that – they limit you and may be undermining your health and holding you back from experiencing the life you desire. It's important that you stop and take a look at your core beliefs because they may be contradicting your goal or vision to be healthy, happy, and living a life that you love.

For example, if deep down you believe that the world is a scary, hostile place and full of people who are out to get you, you will continue to look for evidence and scenarios that support this view and inevitably experience more of it (even if you consciously say that you want more peace). However, if you believe that the world is a kind place, full of loving people who uplift and support each other, you will find evidence of that as well. It's funny because once you shift your belief, the people in your life may not change, but the way you see and interpret them does!

When it comes to health and healing, it's important to look at what you actually believe about who you are, your limitations, your capabilities, who God is, and what you believe about disease, and healing. You can start by asking yourself questions about your beliefs and contemplating the answers. I find it helpful to pray and ask that God reveal to me any subconscious beliefs or anything outside of my awareness that is not aligned with Truth or Love, so that I could heal it and let it go.

Over the years I have identified and upgraded some limiting beliefs that I believe had been significantly blocking my ability to heal. Here is an example. During my breast cancer recovery, I had a strong knowing and desire I needed to identify and remove any subconscious beliefs or programming that contributed to my experience of a decade-long struggle with chronic illness and now cancer. While doing some powerful emotional and spiritual work, I had a vision of the time when I was about five years old and was accidentally severely burned on my legs and hands from hot butter. My grandpa and I were making popcorn in the kitchen and I was sitting on the counter watching him. He slipped a Tupperware dish of butter in the microwave to melt it. When he took it out the bottom collapsed and the sizzling hot butter scorched my legs and hands. Thankfully, my grandpa was a medic in the Army, so he knew to yank off my tights and put me under cold water and rushed me to the hospital. I ended up with third degree burns; however, the medical staff did an incredible job and the scars on my legs are hardly noticeable. This event is actually my first conscious memory. Now back to the vision. I actually saw myself after the fact, during my recovery time, with bandages on my legs and hands, playing a musical instrument my dad had given me. I was happy and smiling. There was no sadness. I was surrounded by my family and seemed to be enjoying the attention. A timeline of my life flashed before me and I saw all the times when I was injured and sick. And then it hit me. Deep down, I had a subconscious belief that was created when I was just a little girl that equated being sick or injured with getting the love and attention I desired. No, it didn't make rational sense, but when we are children we take things quite literal. Tears streamed down my face. I realized that all the love I was seeking was already present within me and that I didn't have to be sick anymore to get it. It was a monumental shift for me and profoundly healing. This belief that was created when I was a child had been drawing experiences of sickness and injury into my life for as long as I've been alive. I was grateful for the awareness and opportunity to upgrade the belief!

Another couple of beliefs that I inherited that I realized were holding me back were that "life is hard" and "I have to work hard to achieve anything worthwhile." When I got sick these beliefs carried over into my quest for healing. I thought that in order to be successful at getting well I had to work really, really, really hard. Unfortunately, this left me exhausted, depleted, always chasing peace and healing, and never really living. The truth is that life's only hard if you believe it's hard. I've met people who flow with life and "roll with the punches." Nothing really seems to fluster them and they seem genuinely joyful. Do you know anyone like this? Ha! I used to be irritated by these people because deep down I wished I could be that way. Now, more and more of the time I am experiencing this life of ease and flow. When a new challenge or perceived stressful situation arises I might default back to that stress response and get stuck in a frenzy with thoughts like "I can't" and "It's too hard," but then I become aware that it's the old program coming up again and I can choose differently. My mantra becomes, "I choose to make this fun and easy" and "I have all the time, energy, and resources I need to accomplish this with ease." My husband often reminds me, "What would it look like if it were easy?" And sure enough, with some breathing and adjustments in thought and feeling I begin to move forward with ease and confidence that I can complete the task without going bonkers. I'm learning to "undo" this program and upgrade this belief into one that is more aligned with the life I want to experience.

Based on my experience, research, and inner knowing I've come to realize that upgrading my beliefs about God, life, health/disease, my limitations, and my capabilities have been powerful catalysts in my healing and living a life of greater ease, love, joy, connection, and freedom. I invite you to take a moment to compare and contrast the two belief systems and the results I experienced from believing in these ways about God, life, health/disease, and myself. Which one is more conducive to healing, wholeness, and joy? What are your beliefs about God, life, health/disease, and yourself? Take some time to contemplate this.

Old, Limiting Belief:

I grew up believing in an impersonal God that exists in the sky somewhere and that if I was "good" enough that I'd earn his favor. I believed that I was never quite good enough and had to work hard, to please, to perform, and to be perfect to get the love and attention that I was seeking. I believed that disease happened as a result of me doing something wrong and being a failure of some kind. I believed that one day I could find that "peace that passes all understanding" and the joy and connection and fulfillment I'd been chasing, but I believed I had to somehow earn it or do enough of the right things. I wanted to believe that I could heal, but I didn't believe in the power within me to do it. I believed if I researched enough, found the right healer, herb, potion, or treatment or the right combination and tried hard enough at it I would heal.

The Result:

The result of these beliefs was a woman who was exhausted and depleted from so many years of trying to be perfect, but never quite measuring up. At her core she felt that she was lacking and wasn't worthy of being loved just as she was. She felt a sense of being separate and disconnected from God despite the regular church attendance, memorized scriptures, and being a "good" person. The internal clamor of her voice wanting to be heard, her heart wanting to authentically express, and her creativity wanting to be unleashed steadily intensified over the years until there was a full-system breakdown. I didn't love myself and I didn't trust myself. And despite saying I knew God, I didn't really ... only in the limited way the intellect can grasp the concept. Although always chasing happiness and fulfillment, I never found it. My body seemed to be chronically sick and no matter how hard I tried I didn't feel well.

New, Life-Affirming Belief:

God, Source, or Divine Intelligence is Love. He is present everywhere, in all things, and is the Creator of all that is. I am a divine manifestation and unique expression of God. The power of the Divine is not outside of me, but is within me and therefore the power that created me can heal me. And if the power of God is within me, it's also in you and therefore I am connected to you and all of Life. I do not inherit disease, nor does God punish me by making me sick. In a spiritual sense I am already whole and in a human sense I am always moving toward a state of wholeness. I trust that I am always loved, supported, and guided. All the love that I was once seeking is already inside of me. I don't have to earn it or hustle for it. This Love is me. Instead of trying to figure it all out on my own, I can listen to the voice of God within me to guide me. I can choose to surrender and flow with Life and it's in my highest good to do so.

The Result:

I am now a woman who, more often than not, feels whole. I love my life and I'm learning to love myself and others in deeper and more intimate ways. The "peace that passes all understanding" is a choice away and my life is full of much more joy, fulfillment, connection, and a sense of freedom than I've never known. I'm learning to express myself authentically, explore my creativity, to flow with life instead of fix or force, to trust and surrender. I know who I am as a beloved child of God – imperfectly perfect, human and divine. I know that I am here to let my light shine, to be of service, and am capable of more than I realize. I still get scared, I still fall down, I still face challenges, and I continue to grow, but for the first time in my life I'm truly living. I'm living full out, loving deeply, and committed to doing so for as long as I am alive.

I share this with you so that you may see what's possible for you and how letting go of my limiting beliefs and upgrading my beliefs about God, life, health/disease, my capabilities, and my limitations has been absolutely essential on my path to healing and wholeness. The key here is to become aware of the limiting beliefs in your life and begin to cultivate life-affirming or empowering beliefs that align with Truth and your vision for your health and life.

In addition to the old and new scenarios I shared, here are a few common beliefs that you may have that may need some exploring and upgrading:

- Limiting: I am a victim of my life situation or this disease.
- Life-affirming: I am a master creator of my reality and I have within me the power to heal. This health challenge is an opportunity for radical growth and transformation.

- Limiting: God must be punishing me because I am not well.
- Life-affirming: God is Love and Love does not punish.

- Limiting: This disease has the power to destroy, harm, or kill me.

- Life-affirming: I am a child of God and I am eternal. The power that created the Universe is also in me and can heal me.

- Limiting: I am not worthy of love.
- Life-affirming: I am worthy of love because love is what I am.

- Limiting: I am not enough.
- Life-affirming: I am enough exactly as I am. I am imperfectly perfect. I am human and divine at the same time.

- Limiting: I don't deserve to be well or happy.
- Life-affirming: I deserve vibrant health, wholeness, peace, and joy because I am a child of God.

- Limiting: Healing myself is hard.
- Life-affirming: I can heal with ease and confidence. I trust in the power within me to heal me. Everything I need to know or do will be revealed to me.

Beliefs about Disease

We live in a world that is dominated by the fear of disease. Chronic illness is escalating and the efforts to fight against these illnesses are in full force. So, why then do these illnesses continue to rise despite all of our efforts? So much money has been raised to fight against cancer and other illnesses, yet we still have people suffering in mass quantities. Is it possible that our individual and collective beliefs about disease are contributing to this epidemic? We seem to believe more in the power of disease to kill and harm than we do in our own power to heal. Currently, the collective consciousness and underlying belief about disease seems to be that it's not a matter of if you will get some disease, but when. Most of us, whether we realize it or not, spend most of our lives programmed by media, culture, and life experiences to fear disease (and death). Is it this fear and belief that getting a disease is just a matter of time that makes us most susceptible to it? Is it this fear that robs us of our peace, joy, and ability to live our lives fully? I don't have all the answers, but it's something to contemplate. Belief is a very powerful thing.

When we view ourselves as physical beings only, it's understandable to see our shortcomings. But, when we realize and believe that we are spiritual beings with human bodies that were meant to thrive and deserve to be well and whole – it changes things. Instead of focusing so much energy and fear on the power of disease to kill and destroy, we choose to focus on the divine power we hold within us to heal and be well, I believe it could help the world to heal and alleviate much suffering.

It Runs in My Family

I've worked with a lot of people struggling with their health. I can't tell you how many times I've heard people blame their illness on their genetics. "It runs in my family," they would say. They believed they had little to no hope in being able to overcome their illness. Sadly, we've been conditioned to believe that much of our health is beyond our control. This is one of the most damaging beliefs that exists. The truth is that most chronic disease is environmental. As mentioned earlier, when it comes to cancer, for example, 5-10% of cancer is genetic, the rest comes from environment and lifestyle factors.[12] The good news about this is that we have more control over our health than we realize!

We know through the study of epigenetics that while we may be genetically predisposed to certain disease conditions, there are *many* biological mechanisms that influence whether particular genes are expressed or not. These mechanisms can switch genes on and off, making them active or dormant based on factors *within our control*, such as what we choose to eat, lifestyle choices, toxin exposure, the interactions we have with others, exercise, and our emotional and mental states (all of which we will explore in this book).

Stem cell biologist and author of *Biology of Belief,* Bruce Lipton, PhD, states: "The difference between these two [genetic determinism and epigenetics] is significant because this fundamental belief called genetic determinism literally means that our lives, which are defined as our physical, physiological, and emotional behavioral traits, are controlled by the genetic code. This kind of belief system provides a visual picture of people being victims: If the genes control our life function, then our lives are being controlled by things outside of our ability to change them. This leads to victimization that the illnesses and diseases that run in families are propagated through the passing of genes associated with those attributes. Laboratory evidence shows this is not true."[13]

Your genetics are not necessarily set in stone. The choices you make about how you live, think, feel, eat, move, and what you believe all play a role in what you experience in your life! Knowing what choices to make can be a bit overwhelming and that's why it's so helpful to have someone to guide you. These are the types of things I cover and help support women with in my coaching program.

Create Awareness

Your thoughts and beliefs are extraordinarily powerful! They can limit you or they can empower you. Begin to create awareness around your thoughts and only choose those thoughts you wish to experience. Consider incorporating meditation into your daily morning practice in order to create more awareness in your mind, and to reap the many health benefits! Also consider using any of the suggestions mentioned to become more aware of the thoughts you are thinking.

What beliefs do you have that aren't aligned with your vision for your health? Be willing to inquire about your deeply held core beliefs so that you can become aware of any faulty programs that are undermining your health and vision. Begin to dismantle beliefs that no longer serve you and upgrade them into ones that are life-affirming and align with the Truth of who you are, your dreams of vibrant health, and living a life you love.

Know that dismantling limiting beliefs can be a process, like peeling back the layers of an onion. But, by having the intention and prayer to become aware of any and all things that are holding you back, those things that need to be released will come to the surface of your awareness so that you can let them go.

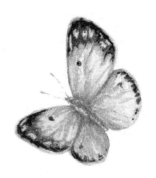

Chapter 6:

Essential #4 –
Feel Your Feelings

*"Since emotions run every system of your body, don't underestimate
their power to contribute to health and disease."*
– Candace Pert, PhD, neuroscientist, author of *Molecules of Emotion*

After spending eight years focusing my healing efforts on my physical body – diet, lifestyle, and supplement programs and protocols – and then getting cancer, I knew in my heart that there was an underlying emotional component that was contributing to my health problems. But, I didn't really know much more than that or what to do about it. I didn't know much about dealing with my emotions. I was never taught how to feel my feelings and effectively manage or address them. Were you? Most likely, not. And I was never taught how important it was for my health and well-being to know how to do this. This is something that only recently has come to my attention. I began to ask God to show me what I needed to know. I prayed that all toxicity in mind, body, heart, and spirit be removed and that if there was anything I needed to know or do on my part that it would be revealed.

Inevitably, certain people, healers, and books came across my path to help me begin to do what I call the "heartwork" necessary to release my faulty mental patterns, beliefs, and suppressed and repressed emotions. After working with some amazing practitioners and using many of the tools I share in this chapter, I became aware of, and continue to work through, much unprocessed and unfelt grief, anger, fear, and resentment that accumulated over a lifetime. Doing so has been essential to the healing of my physical body, and much to my surprise, has allowed me to feel a deeper sense of peace, ease, spiritual connection, joy, and freedom that I had been seeking my whole life. A whole new way of living and enjoying my life began to open. Through this process I've also learned how to feel my feelings and manage my emotions in my day-to-day experience so that I don't continue to stuff these emotions and cause harm to my body, mind, and spirit. I can't emphasize how important and powerful addressing my emotions has been (and continues to be) in my healing journey.

Through my own experience, research, and working with other women struggling with their health, I've learned that when it comes to chronic disease there is always an emotional component. This is one of the *most* overlooked pieces of the puzzle when it comes to health. Recall that you are a dynamic, holistic being with a physical, mental, emotional, and spiritual body. To heal, you must address all bodies – not just the physical. Learning to effectively deal with your emotions on a daily basis, as well as heal emotional wounds from the past are key elements to your emotional well-being.

We've already touched a bit on the power of our feeling state. In Chapter 4, we discussed the creative power of thoughts, words, and feelings and how we can use them to harness our ability to heal by aligning them with our vision. We know that thoughts + feelings go hand in hand and that by combining an intention with an elevated emotional state we can positively and powerfully influence our environment and our bodies! You learned how the stress or "fight or flight" response is activated through our thinking and feeling. When we chronically feel depleting emotions such as fear, anxiety, or worry, the body stays in this "fight or flight" stressful state, which causes it to become out of balance and prone to physical illness. Needless to say, our emotions are *powerful* drivers of our physiology, physical health, overall well-being, and our ability to create the life experiences we desire.

The Nature of Emotions

What exactly are emotions? The nature of emotions has historically been a tricky thing to fully grasp and define, but we do know they are an essential part of our day-to-day life experiences and the quality of those experiences. The word "emotion" is derived from the Latin word "emotere," which means "energy in motion." I like this because it reminds us that emotions are meant to move versus staying stuck or stagnant!

Emotions, just like thoughts, are energy and according to neuroscientist Candace Pert, PhD, are the bridges or the unifying elements between body and mind, which we once previously believed were separate entities. Her research revealed that neuropeptides or the "molecules of emotion" run every system of the body and demonstrate the intelligence of this unified "bodymind," making emotions more important than we thought when it comes to our overall health and well-being. Pert explains this further when she states, "The chemicals that are running our body and our brain are the same chemicals that are involved in emotion. And that says to me that we'd better pay more attention to emotions with respect to health."[14]

More and more researchers and healers are beginning to realize the importance of emotions when it comes to being and staying well. I'm tellin' ya ... emotions are important, y'all!

We each experience a symphony of emotions on a daily basis – some of the most common ones being sadness, anger, happiness, fear, and excitement. Feeling is an integral part of the human experience that brings meaning, contrast, and texture to our lives. No matter how hard we try we cannot successfully stop feeling (although to our detriment we try). However, we can become better equipped at moving through challenging emotions, managing our emotional energy, and learning to activate renewing and healing emotions to invite deeper levels of healing, peace, and joy in our lives.

Many of us are quick to label certain feelings as bad and expend a great deal of energy wanting to avoid them or stuff them. Feelings such as sadness, anger, and fear are often labeled as "negative." But these emotions are all a part of what it means to be human and these feelings enrich and expand our lives in countless ways. For example, the experience of feeling sad about something can lead to compassion for others. Or have you ever gone through a time when you felt sad for several days? How much more were you able to appreciate the joyful moments having had experienced the contrast of sadness? Anger can make us realize that a different course of action needs to take place and inspire us to do it, which leads to greater happiness. Fear can keep us safe from harm. These emotions aren't bad, they are part of the intricate web of our emotional experience as human beings. Emotions, just like thoughts, are part of who we are as humans – but it's helpful to remember that our thoughts and feelings aren't who we are at our essence or spiritual core. Although it doesn't always seem to be the case, you actually can have dominion over your thinking and feeling world. You don't always have to be at the mercy of your emotions and in state of overwhelm and attachment with your thoughts. Learning how to do this takes becoming more aware, emotionally intelligent, and improving your ability to manage your energy, which are all things that I emphasize and focus on in my program.

Emotional Intelligence

It's not about getting rid of your emotions (because we can't), denying them, ignoring them, wallowing in them, or swallowing them

… it's about gaining awareness about them, feeling them, and being able to choose how we will respond versus allowing them to take over and run the show. These are core elements of emotional intelligence. Our culture and educational system emphasize the diligent sharpening and expansion of our intellectual intelligence, but it doesn't pay much attention to teaching us emotional intelligence, which is arguably just as important or more so than IQ in our success, quality of life, and health. The majority of us are ill equipped to deal with our emotions, and it's time for us all to begin learning to cultivate our emotional skills and understanding in order to be well, happier, and more at peace in the world!

What exactly is emotional intelligence, you may be wondering? Emotional intelligence has to do with your ability to identify and manage your emotions and the emotions of others effectively. Daniel Goleman, author of *Emotional Intelligence: Why It Can Matter More than IQ*, identifies four aspects of emotional intelligence which include self-awareness (being able to identify your emotions and emotions of others), self-management (being able to handle or manage those emotions effectively or being emotionally resilient), empathy (being able to know what someone else is feeling), and social skills (being able to put it all together in relationships with people). Emotional intelligence requires practice and cultivation and it starts with self-awareness and being willing to feel your feelings.

Feel Your Feelings

Self-awareness involves checking in with yourself and being able to identify what you are feeling. It takes practice to become more aware of what you are feeling, because most people aren't used to or taught to do so. Meditation and mindfulness practices are helpful tools to cultivate self-awareness. It's important and extremely beneficial to take time for quiet and solitude to be able to check in with your emotions. Just learning the simple act of checking in daily and asking, "What do I feel?" can be incredibly helpful in learning to become more emotionally intelligent. Consider taking multiple one to five minute peace periods throughout the day where you step away from the hustle and bustle of the day, get still, connect with and slow down your breathing, and check in with how you are feeling.

In each coaching session that I have with my clients I have them check in with how they are feeling in their emotional body before we begin. It's not uncommon for a woman to struggle at first with being able to name her feelings, but over time it gets easier as she becomes more practiced and connected with her body and emotions. It's also not uncommon for a woman to be thrown off guard when emotions come bubbling to the surface that she didn't know she had once she took the space and time to get still and check in with herself.

Your emotions and body are connected. Recall how you feel "butter-flies" in your stomach when you are nervous or perhaps you feel heat in your chest when you are angry. Your body will give you clues to how you are feeling emotionally. This is why it can be helpful to do a body scan to help you get in touch with your emotions.

Here's how to do a body scan:

Find a comfortable place to sit or lay down. Close your eyes and use your attention to scan your body from the top of your head to the bottoms of your feet. If you notice any tension or restriction in your physical body or any sadness, anger, fear, or frustration that arises, just be with it for a moment without judgment. Feel it, breathe deeply, and let whatever you are feeling be okay. Sometimes tears come up. Let them fall. Take a moment to breathe into any areas of tension and consciously relax them, which also can be a helpful way to move stagnant energy.

In addition to getting in the habit of checking in with yourself and asking how you feel, it's important to now give yourself full permission to feel all your feelings without labeling them as "good" or "bad." All feelings are meant to be felt, touched with love (even the so-called "negative" ones) and moved. Remember, emotional energy is meant to move fluidly throughout the body. Most of us resist the unwanted feelings like fear or sadness and try to push them away. This does no good. I've said it before and I'll say it again – what you resist persists. The magic that transforms the sadness into your joy, for example, begins with accepting and allowing the sadness and touching it with love. It is acceptance and love that will transform those uncomfortable and often painful feelings. Resisting, avoiding, ignoring, stuffing, or suppressing emotions does no good, only causes more pain and discomfort, and creates blockages of energy in the body. But where does this stagnant energy go? Karol Truman wrote a book that sums up the answer entitled *Feelings Buried Alive Never Die*. These lower vibration emotions, such as fear and grief, that you don't want or know how to feel stay stuck and stress the systems of your body unless you feel and move them. When you chronically and repeatedly suppress your emotions it impairs the functioning of the physical body. Chronic emotional distress, angst, and fear negatively impact the immune system and the body's ability to effectively regulate inflammation, which increases risk for many physical ailments and diseases including cancer.[15]

Once you identify what you are feeling and allow yourself to feel it, consider incorporating techniques that may help to move the energy. Because of this connection between body and emotion, doing things that move your physical body or get energy moving in your body can be very beneficial. Incorporating things like dancing (especially combined with music), exercising, breath work, massage, and energy work (reiki, acupuncture, etc.) can be helpful ways to process emotions and keep emotional energy flowing. We will talk more about other helpful tools to move and process emotions later in this chapter.

To recap, it's essential to welcome and feel all emotions and love what arises without judgment. Being willing to love even the "negative emotions" will allow you to dissolve that energy and transform it into renewing or positive emotional energy. The energy of love always heals. Keep in mind, you don't necessarily want to let your feelings take you over and attach or identify with them, which is where emotional intelligence and energy management comes in.

Energy Management

In addition to being aware of your emotions, it's important to be able to effectively manage them in order to experience a sense of wellness, reduce stress, have healthy relationships, and be successful in all areas of your life. Being able to effectively manage emotional energy in everyday life experiences and encounters has to do with being resilient and being able to regulate your emotional responses. Resilience is the ability to overcome and effectively adapt in the face of challenging situations.

Have you ever gotten so angry in the moment that you said some things you didn't mean to someone you cared about that forever changed the quality of your relationship? Or perhaps you lashed out at work and lost your job or suffered negative consequences because of it? Have you experienced times when you were feeling immense sadness for days on end, all the while forcing a smile and telling everyone you are "great"? Perhaps you avoided and denied the sadness and kept it all in, but the truth was that you felt miserable and it was affecting your job, your health, marriage, and relationship with your kids. You didn't know what to do about it, so you kept it inside and tried to hide it from everyone else. This overwhelming feeling of depression likely came from layers and layers of unfelt, unexpressed emotions and now it's impacting every part of your life. These are just a few examples of how not being able to effectively process and regulate your emotions can affect your life.

Being able to manage your emotional energy and learning to be resilient in the face of challenges is a critical skill, not only for your happiness, quality of life, success in your professional life and relationships, but most importantly for your health and overcoming chronic illness. One study of over five thousand middle-aged people with chronic disease demonstrated that those with the highest self-regulation ability were *fifty times* more likely to be alive and without chronic disease fifteen years later.[16]

This is so important! And it's important to realize these are skills that we learn, which is why I place a huge focus on energy management in my coaching program. It never fails: as my clients begin to become more effective at managing their emotional energy, they start to sound and look so much lighter and experience more well-being in their lives.

Heart Coherence

In addition to meditation and mindfulness techniques to assist with cultivating more emotional intelligence, resilience, and improved energy management, I recommend using HeartMath tools and technologies. These are powerful tools that I use consistently on a day-to-day basis, as well as with my clients, in order to cultivate heart coherence, become more effective at self-regulating emotions, and improve the ability to handle stressful situations as they arise. Because stress is such a key factor in all illness, I've found these tools to be some of the most helpful for all women dealing with chronic illness.

We touched on heart coherence in Chapter 4, but I want to review and dive into more here. Heart coherence is an optimal state of functioning that synchronizes the heart and mind and creates harmony in the systems of the body. Being in a state of coherence is associated with improvements in health, performance, and overall well-being. HeartMath Institute Research Director Rolling McCraty describes coherence this way: "Coherence is the state when the heart, mind and emotions are in energetic alignment and cooperation. It is a state that builds resiliency – personal energy is accumulated, not wasted – leaving more energy to manifest intentions and harmonious outcomes."[17] Guess what drives this coherent state? You guessed it! Emotion – specifically positive or elevated emotional states. Remember in Chapter 4 how the HeartMath study demonstrated that power of thought or intention combined with being in a coherent state was able to unwind strands of DNA? The process through which we access this coherent state is through connecting with the heart. It involves slowing down the breath and breathing in and out of the heart, combined with the activation of positive, core emotions of the heart such as love, gratitude, care, and compassion. The more you practice being in a coherent state, the more you are able to benefit and the better you are able to self-regulate your emotions.

Studies conducted by the HeartMath Institute have demonstrated that one's emotional state can be consistently reflected through observing heart rate variability or heart rhythms. When a person is in what is called an incoherent state (fueled by depleting emotions such as fear, frustration, anxiety, and worry), the visual result on the heart rate variability monitor displays a jagged, inconsistent heart rhythm (see Figure 1). In this state, the heart is sending chaotic signals to the brain and your ability to think clearly and process information is impaired. When you are in this incoherent state you are draining your energy reserves. When this happens consistently and chronically you experience those negative effects of prolonged stress, which include weakening of immunity, hormone imbalance, a variety of physical ailments, and ultimately disease.

When a person is in a coherent state (activating love, gratitude, and care) the heart rate variability pattern is a smooth, consistent, sinusoidal wave as shown in Figure 1. Being in a state of coherence helps the body to function more efficiently with less energy required. It helps to improve overall health and well-being and has been shown to improve the following: ability to access your inner guidance or intuition, sleep, ability to handle and recover from stress, reaction times, mental clarity, performance, creativity, memory, focus, and learning.[18]

Figure 1

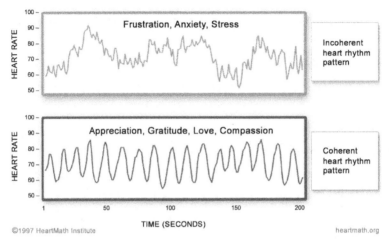

Image courtesy of the HeartMath Institute – www.heartmath.org

For any woman dealing with chronic illness, the ability to reduce stress and become more emotionally resilient is absolutely paramount to healing. Not to mention, learning to get into a coherent state allows you to better access the wisdom of your heart and intuition. Being able to follow your inner guidance is of the upmost importance in making health and life decisions for your highest and best good (more about this in Chapter 11).

Quick Coherence Technique®

The Quick Coherence Technique® is a super quick and easy Heart-Math tool that you can use to get into a state of coherence. You can do it anytime, anywhere, with eyes open or closed! Keep in mind that it's the elevated *feeling* that creates coherence. The more often you are in a coherent state, the better you are able to regulate and manage your energy, recharge your inner battery, be more resilient in the face of adversity, and experience the many benefits previously mentioned.

Here are the steps for the HeartMath Quick Coherence Technique®:

Step 1:

Heart-Focused Breathing

Focus your attention in the area of the heart. Imagine your breath is flowing in and out of your heart or chest area, breathing a little slower and deeper than usual.

Suggestion: Inhale 5 seconds, exhale 5 seconds (or whatever rhythm is comfortable).

Step 2:

Activate a Positive Feeling

Make a sincere attempt to experience a regenerative feeling such as appreciation or care for someone or something in your life.

Suggestion: Try to re-experience the feeling you have for someone you love, a pet, a special place, an accomplishment, etc. or focus on a feeling of calm or ease.

Emotions powerfully influence much of our thinking, bodily processes, and the quality of our everyday life experiences. You may have been told when you were feeling down to just "think good thoughts" or say positive affirmations aloud. These can be helpful things, but if you are trying to think and say positive things but your feeling state is in direct opposition, you will likely not have much luck getting happy. However, getting in tune with and fully feeling the underlying emotion and then activating a coherent state through elevated emotions often creates harmony in the mind as well.

The emotions we feel dictate the stress we experience in mind and body, influence decisions, motivate your actions, affect your judgment, direct your attention, and effect your memory and learning processes. This has profound effects on your quality of life and your health. Thoughts are important, but it is through accessing states of coherence via elevated emotional states and breathing slowly in and out of the heart that we can take advantage of the power of the heart to improve overall healing and well-being.

Recap

I know that was quite a bit of information, so in case you missed anything here's a quick overview of tips to improve emotional intelligence:

1. Create more awareness about how you are feeling
   - Check in with how you are feeling daily or throughout the day
   - Do a body scan
   - Meditation/mindfulness
2. Give yourself full permission to feel your feelings
3. Avoid labeling your feelings as good or bad
4. Allow and love whatever emotions arise
5. Move your body and/or incorporate techniques to move energy and process emotions
6. Activate heart coherence to shift your emotional state, reduce stress, and improve your ability to manage your energy

Healing Emotional Wounds

If you truly want to heal your body and live a life that you love you must be willing to heal your emotional wounds. I cannot emphasize this enough. As mentioned before, every woman with chronic illness likely has an emotional component to the disease they are experiencing. Often these emotional wounds experienced from a one-time event from the past have reverberating effects for years and even a lifetime in ways you don't realize. Unexpressed or repressed pain, grief, or resentment experienced from this event gets stored in the body and can be replayed over and over in the mind, further perpetuating the damage and disease in mind, body, heart, and spirit.

It's important to understand that it's not just about trying to feel positive emotions all the time when it comes to healing. Yes, creating positive thinking and feeling states daily is a powerful tool to improve your well-being and tap into your co-creative power. However, don't forget the importance of taking time to feel whatever feelings arise in the moment, including sadness, anger, or fear, as well as taking the time to address the stored up, stockpiled pain and wounds from the past. According to Dr. Pert, "All honest emotions are positive emotions." Choosing to feel and heal suppressed anger or resentment can bolster the immune system and be a catalyst for deep healing.[19]

Releasing and dissolving emotional wounds takes courage, vulnerability, and can take time. Like shedding limiting beliefs, it can be like peeling back layers of an onion and is rarely a quick fix. One layer will surface to be felt and healed and then the next layer is primed and ready when the time is right. Committing to healing your emotional wounds isn't always easy but so worth it. So many women would much rather keep things buried than actually feel them, even if it is the very thing necessary to help them fully heal their physical body.

I had a potential client that I was on the phone with discussing whether or not it would be a good fit to work together. After a brief discussion, I knew she had many layers of emotional wounds that were likely causing much disease and disharmony in her body and life. I explained that part of my program was to begin to look at how emotions play a role in health. I could tell she was reluctant. She told me about a time when she tried out a yoga class that involved some breath work. While she was doing the breathing exercises, she started to cry uncontrollably and it scared her. She left the class. The breath and crying are ways the body releases and cleanses stored emotional energy. Her body needed to purge. This was a very healing thing that was happening. I told her this, but she was clear that she didn't want to explore any past emotional hurts. Unfortunately, as much as she wanted to feel better, she wasn't ready to have anything to do with looking at her emotions and how they were impacting her health.

Many women are so afraid to feel their feelings because we were never taught how to, encouraged to, felt safe enough to do so, and perhaps we were even reprimanded or told not to "be emotional." Emotionality has taken on a negative connotation and implies weakness in our society, further encouraging us to run away from our feelings and the storms of life. What an unfortunate and misguided belief that I recommend we all unsubscribe to!

Be Like the Buffalo

I heard this story once about the difference between how cows and buffalo respond to storms and I think it's a helpful metaphor when it comes to dealing with emotional turmoil and the storms of life. Like most of us, when cows sense a storm coming they begin moving in the opposite direction to flee from the storm. However, when buffalo sense a storm coming they begin moving directly into it. Guess which one gets stuck in the storm longer and experiences more suffering as a result? The cows. Because the cows aren't very fast the storm catches up to them, often intensifies in the process, and follows them as they both move in the same direction. The cows end up spending more time in the bad weather and experience more struggle. The buffalo, however, move through the storm faster by going into it and end up experiencing less suffering along the way.

When it comes to the emotional wounds of the past and the perceived unpleasant emotions that arise in the moment, be like the buffalo – go into it. I understand that you may have resistance and fear to drudging up the old stuff. It's uncomfortable at first, and even painful when choosing to feel unpleasant feelings from the past. But in order to heal and to live a life of peace and well-being the only way is to move through it so it can be released and transformed. There is so much glorious freedom on the other side of liberating those toxic feelings that have been brewing inside of you for ages.

Letting Your Fear Speak

Living in a state of fear keeps us stuck and blocks us from accessing our heart and our healing power within. We know this and so when we feel fear we try to outrun it, hide, and push it away in a panic, but usually these tactics don't work and it continues to stick around and make us feel like we are suffocating. It's incapacitating. Fear is one of what Louise Hay calls the "Big Four" in her book, *The Power is Within You*, along with resentment, criticism, and guilt and describes them as the biggest things that hold us back in our lives.

Do we want to live in perpetual fear and make decisions from a place of fear? No! We understand the negative impact that staying in a state of chronic stress and fear has on the body and mind. And because we know this, we become afraid of fear itself and try to dodge and avoid it, which only invites more of it. The truth is that we all feel fear. Fear is inevitable. So, what if you shift the way you relate to fear? Instead of trying to push it away, consider thinking of fear as a friend. I know it sounds a little crazy, but fear can (if you let it) be a guide, nudging you back to the truth of who you are – Love. When you feel fear, instead of pushing the fear away I invite you to feel the fear fully. Remember, all honest emotions are positive ones. Feel it in your body. Where is it? Does it have a color? A shape? Breathe into it. Ask it what it is trying to tell you and then listen. Let it be heard and thank it for its concern. And once the fear is heard and felt it creates an opportunity and opening for it to be transformed.

Fear transforms into faith once we touch it with love, feel it, and let it speak. It may be helpful to get out a piece of paper and dump all fears on the paper. Give it a voice. It is staying stuck in the fear that keeps us prisoners in our own minds and causes disharmony in the body. But, when fear arises and we give ourselves permission to feel it and have the courage to acknowledge it, and listen to it instead of hiding from it, it moves through us and we are able to return to a place of love.

Anger – No More "I'm Fine"

Beloved, I give you full permission to be angry and to express that anger. It's time. Your health depends on it. You've been holding it in and sugarcoating this raw emotion far too long. In our culture, sadness – gentle weeping and sullen expressions – are acceptable. Expression of anger by women – yelling and screaming and stomping of feet – is not. It's not "lady-like," you see. We grew up in families and in a society where it wasn't acceptable or encouraged to express anger. We've been gulping down our anger for years, faking smiles and offering platitudes like "I'm fine," when asked how we are feeling. We dare not express our anger. How many times have you said you were "fine" in your lifetime, all the while seething and bubbling beneath the surface? Where do the years and years of pent up molten hot anger go?

Anger that's been stuffed down and bottled up turns to resentment or depression that eats away at you like a parasite. As you now know, it creates disease in the body. It's time to delete "fine" from your vocabulary. It's time to feel the anger and learn to express it in healthy ways. Have you ever watched an infant have a temper tantrum? She cries and wails and stomps or writhes around on the ground because she's angry she can't have her way. Within minutes she's smiling and enthralled with a new toy. The anger is there, she feels it, and she moves through it rather quickly. As adults, we get angry too and we need to express it. I'm not saying you should throw a temper tantrum in the grocery store because they are out of stock of your favorite gluten-free crackers, but you need to learn to *move* your anger in a healthy and positive way that doesn't hurt other people. Sometimes we need to beat some pillows, go for a run, scream and yell out loud or into a pillow, or stomp the ground in the privacy of our own homes. I have a whole "Angry" music playlist. I like to dance it out by myself in my living room or with some girlfriends. The angry music brings my anger to the surface to help me feel it. Music has a way of moving emotional energy in the body. Moving your body to the music; stomping, kicking, punching, writhing on the floor, yelling, and sweating can all help me to move that energy. Try it! You'll feel like a new woman afterwards. Free therapy in your living room! I highly recommend it.

To some of you this sounds incredibly embarrassing and you are extremely reluctant and maybe even resistant to doing this. I have to admit, expressing my anger through dancing, screaming, and punching pillows was a little awkward and embarrassing at first – even though I was alone. I was being asked to forego the poise and the "cool, calm, collected, keep it all together" persona that I had been trained to maintain at all times. However, I must say once I got out of my head and gave myself permission to feel the feelings in my body it was a transformative experience. It felt amazing and so much lighter!

As you begin to flex your feeling muscles and practice expressing your anger, you may have outbursts and ruffle a few feathers. You can't please everyone all the time. I remember the first time I expressed my anger to Chad about something. It was only in the past couple years that I realized I had been repressing my anger and I couldn't do it any longer. I was the queen of "I'm fine" – always holding my tongue and refraining from speaking my truth. No more.

Chad and I had been having several disagreements about something related to work (we were working together at the time) and I was really angry about the way he was handling things. One day he noticed my energy was off and asked me if I was okay. My first automatic reply of "I'm fine" began to slip through my lips, but I stopped it. I paused. I took a breath and I unleashed the rage that had been building for weeks. I told him how angry I was. I yelled and I screamed and I cried. I admit, it was over the top, but I think I was actually releasing years of pent up anger that was totally unrelated to this particular issue. He took a step back and stared back at me with wide eyes. He hadn't witnessed me express my anger. Ever. There was a thick, heavy silence and then he got angry and yelled back. Did I say some things a bit harshly? Yes. And had I processed this on my own first I would've been able to express my anger in a more calm and loving way without saying hurtful things to him. But, I was learning a new skill. I asked Chad to forgive me and I forgave myself. I don't regret it one bit, because it felt a heck of a lot better to express myself than to keep it all in. We laugh about it now. I have since learned to channel and address my anger through things like dancing, talking to a trusted friend, journaling, meditation, essential oils, and other techniques. And if after that I still feel called to have a conversation with someone, I will, and I am able to do it from a loving, calm place.

Another way to express your anger is simply to share your anger honestly and openly with the person you feel angry with. For example, if Chad said something that angered me, instead of lashing out, I take the space I need to process my emotions. I dance it out or go for a walk and then I ask to speak with him. From this place, I am able to share my feelings in a calm, non-reactive state. We are then able to work it out without screaming at each other. I'm becoming much more effective at managing my energy.

Anger transforms into authority. The energy of anger can be refining and sharpening. It can be used for fueling positive change and taking ownership and authority in your life. It also transforms into forgiveness. However, when it's stuffed down, stuck, and smoldering, it leads to resentment and depression. Anger has gotten a bad rap. Both men *and* women alike feel anger all the time. It's okay to feel angry. Give yourself permission to feel it and use constructive techniques to move that anger into a more empowered version of yourself. Move and express the anger and then forgive. Always forgive, let it go, and move on. Save the word "fine" to describe china or dining – not as a cover-up for what's truly going on underneath the surface.

Grief

We all experience grief, but unfortunately, we aren't very well prepared to deal with it. It is a normal and natural part of living and arises when there is loss or change of any kind. Whether it's a death of a loved one or pet, loss of a relationship, divorce, moving to a new place or starting a new job and leaving the old behind, or even loss of trust or safety – all can be a catalyst for feeling grief. According to *The Grief Recovery Handbook*, grief is a neglected and misunderstood process in which we are socialized to attempt to resolve grief with our intellect or heads versus our hearts, which ultimately leads to failure to fully resolve it.

Are you holding on to unresolved grief from the past? Unresolved grief is a huge stressor on your body, mind, and spirit. It can be a massive energy drain that if not felt or resolved can make you sick, hold you back from healing, negatively impact your relationships and job, and keep you feeling stuck. Perhaps you can identify losses in your life that stick out to you in which your heart was broken. Were you able to fully grieve that situation or person? It's likely that you did not have the tools to properly do so and it's not your fault. Being encouraged and taught how to feel our feelings in general, including how to grieve, is not something we were taught growing up. If you suspect there is an event from your past that you have not fully grieved that could be negatively impacting your health, I recommend working with a practitioner that can help you move through your grief, help you to see how this grief has affected your life, and help you to deal with related unresolved emotions. The Grief Recovery Method is an excellent program to help you do this and you can find groups and practitioners in your area and online.

Feeling Good

As we've discussed in previous chapters, it is your feeling state that drives your physiology and can put you into a state of "fight or flight" or "rest, repair, and rejuvenate." Chronic states of "fight or flight," fear, and stress create disease in the body. Conversely, by invoking positive emotional states such as gratitude combined with heart-focused breathing, we can create coherence or an optimal physiologic state in which the brain, heart, and nervous systems are in sync, the body is able to "rest, repair, and rejuvenate" and is a state that improves overall well-being.

Cultivating daily practices and using tools that activate elevated emotional states helps us feel good and are essential to being well in body, mind, and spirit. However, it's crucial to remember that it's important to first feel the not-so-pleasant feelings when they arise. As we discussed, it's important to touch all feelings with love, allow them, and feel them fully. By doing this you are able to move into an elevated feeling state much easier. Gratitude and forgiveness are two of what I call "superpowers" because they help us achieve states of love, peace, joy, and freedom quickly – especially if we learn to cultivate them as a daily practice.

Gratitude

Gratitude is the springboard back to joy and has the capacity to dig you out of the darkest of times. Let's be honest. When you are dealing with pain, functional limitations, fatigue, and the fear, anger, and sadness that often accompanies illness it's easy to get stuck in a spiral of negativity. Trust me, I've been there. Sometimes it feels impossible to break through to the light, but you know staying stuck in the vortex of negative emotions is only going to make things worse and is not a state conducive to healing. You need a hack to get out of the black hole and that's where gratitude comes in. It's a simple yet powerful tool. I know in times of difficulty, crisis, or illness it may seems impossible to be grateful. But, the reality is that there is always something to be grateful for. Invoking the power of gratitude takes more than "thinking good thoughts" or merely trying to "be more grateful." Gratitude requires the use of the head *and* the activation of the heart.

In the moments of darkness and difficulty, you activate your gratitude superpower by consciously choosing to find and focus with your mind on what you are grateful for. Start small. You can be grateful that your husband bought the soft, fluffy toilet paper instead of the scratchy kind. You can be grateful for the potted geranium on your window sill that you love to look at. You can be grateful for your dog that's always excited to see you when you come home. The possibilities are endless. You then begin to feel appreciation for the gifts in your life and the heart gets involved. Watch how choosing to focus on what you are thankful for and to feel appreciation, your load lightens a bit and the enormity of the fear or sadness begins to subside or fall away altogether. The more you cultivate and practice gratitude, the better you are able to shift your thinking, feelings, and perceptions from negative to positive. Gratitude uplifts, inspires, energizes, connects, heals, and creates. By getting grateful you are raising your vibrational frequency and moving into a state that is more conducive to healing, happiness, and experiencing the life that you dream of having.

In previous chapters, we talked about how thought combined with deep feelings of love and gratitude unleash our co-creative abilities to manifest and create the desires of our hearts. Thinking and imagining your dreams while being in the positive feeling state of appreciation as if your dream has already been fulfilled, sends an electromagnetic signature to the Universe pulling your desires toward you. Spending time daily thinking and imagining yourself vibrant and healthy, feeling the feelings of what it feels like to be healthy, and feeling *gratitude* for your healthy body (as if it's already happening now) is one of the most powerful practices you can do!

Practicing gratitude spills over into all aspects of your life and the following benefits may be experienced as a result:
- improved immunity
- decreased stress levels and improved ability to handle stressful situations or crisis
- improved energy levels
- improved sense of well-being and happiness
- strengthening of relationships and social bonds
- transformation of anger into forgiveness
- transformation of fear into faith and courage
- enhances self-esteem
- better sleep

Three Steps to a Daily Gratitude Practice

Don't just think of gratitude as a superpower you can use in rough patches, but also as a daily practice that when cultivated charges your inner battery and translates into the experience of more joy, peace, and love overall. The more you practice, the more you benefit. I highly recommend making a gratitude practice part of your daily morning practice.

Here are three steps to follow:

1 – Contemplation

Begin the day contemplating and jotting down five things you are truly grateful for. Don't just go through the motions and try to avoid using the same things every day (i.e. husband, dog, house, health, etc.). Be specific. It can be big things or small things. It doesn't matter.

For example:

- "I am grateful for watching the sunrise while I drink my delicious cup of matcha tea."
- "I am grateful for my husband doing the laundry today without my having to ask him."

2 – Thought + Feeling

Breathe in and out of your heart slowly and deeply. Using the five things you've just written down, pick one, and visualize it. Next, let the elevated feeling of gratitude wash over you. Spend a couple minutes with the feeling.

3 – Integration

It's time to extend and expand your gratitude to the people in your life. When you include others in your experience of gratitude, the feeling amplifies and it creates ripples of more gratitude and love in your life and the entire world. You can do this in a few different ways. I recommend visualizing a person whom you are grateful for in your mind's eye and sending him/her virtual gratitude, love, and blessings. You can also extend gratitude by calling them up, telling them in person, or writing them a note. Tell the people in your life how much you love them and how grateful you are for them. Take an opportunity to tell someone how something they did or said meant a lot to you or inspired and uplifted you. You may also choose to express appreciation by a tangible gift or act of service, which is also a beautiful expression of gratitude.

Forgiveness

"Forgiveness is the key to happiness." This is one of the many lessons in *A Course in Miracles* and when I read it I paused for quite a long while to take in the magnitude of the statement. Wouldn't we all love to know the "key" to happiness? I know I would! Happiness is elusive in our culture. If there was a "happy" pill I'm sure we'd all swallow it in a heartbeat. Instead we chase happiness down various rabbit holes which often end in addictions to drugs, alcohol, sex, shopping, social media, or whatever it is for you. But, we never actually find the lasting happiness chasing after these things and instead often experience negative repercussions. Could happiness come from the simple act of consistent and persistent forgiveness? I wondered. I was definitely curious, intrigued, and willing to give it a try. How often do I actually forgive? I thought. I guess I really just reserve forgiveness for those obvious situations when I was really hurt by someone. *Perhaps forgiving more frequently is important,* I thought, and decided to explore further.

I'm guessing if you were like me then forgiveness isn't a daily affair or something you do with consistency. In addition to *A Course in Miracles,* Jesus and many of the great masters taught about the importance of forgiveness. In the Bible Jesus was asked how often to forgive and he responded, "seventy times seven" (Matthew 18:22). I take that to mean that it's important to forgive *a lot* or as much as it takes to be free from the prison of unforgiveness. While I was going through alternative treatments at one of the cancer treatment centers I stayed at, I worked with an incredible man who was a Doctor of Medical Qigong. In addition to the energy sessions he gave me, he highly encouraged me to forgive everyone and everything in my life that there was to forgive. He told me that this was incredibly important in my healing process, so I did it, and it turned out to be extremely healing and powerful for me!

Forgiveness, along with gratitude, is a superpower. It is a key to happiness, as well as inner peace and freedom from fear, and is essential to healing. Forgiveness is even considered the highest form of love! When we hold on to grievances and unforgiveness (even small, petty ones that we often forget about) we allow fear to lurk in our minds and therefore are never in our "right" mind. Unforgiveness – a derivative of fear – closes off our hearts, and sabotages our ability to receive love, abundance, miracles, healing, and the ability to manifest and experience our heart's desires. Unforgiveness becomes a breeding ground for disease in body, mind, and spirit. Harboring unforgiveness in the form of anger and hatred causes chronic anxiety, produces excess cortisol and adrenaline, and chronically stresses and depletes your immune system and entire body. Did you know that unforgiveness is actually referred to as a disease in medical books?!

But, what if you learned to forgive on the spot? Boom. You wouldn't allow those emotions to fester and make you sick.

Forgiveness allows you to let go of the energy suck that keeps you stuck in hoping the past will be any different than what it was. How much energy do you waste wishing things would've been different, holding on to the pain and refusing to forgive? The past is over and there is no sense in wasting time replaying these hurts over and over in your mind. Forgiveness heals and sets you free.

We are always either operating from a place of love or fear. Love is our True Nature and decisions made and actions taken from this place are always aligned to our highest and best good. Therefore, forgiveness not only offers freedom from fear, but allows love to prevail. Healing happens when we are aligned with Love, when we are at peace in our hearts – it is here the divine perfection of our cells, organs, glands, and systems of the body begin to return to harmony. It allows our body's innate healing ability to activate.

Daily Forgiveness Inventory

Choosing to forgive past hurts (more about this in Chapter 9), as well as making forgiveness a daily practice is extraordinarily powerful when it comes to healing, inner peace, and well-being. Being able to forgive in the moment is tremendously valuable and takes a certain level of emotional intelligence, mindfulness, and practice. We are constantly experiencing emotions throughout our day-to-day experiences and interactions with people. There's not always time to process feelings in the moment. Therefore, it's an excellent practice at the end of the day to take some time to be alone with yourself and do a forgiveness inventory. It's an act of cleansing your emotional body. It is so simple, but don't underestimate how important and powerful this can be!

Here's how:

Before bed find a quiet place where you can be uninterrupted. You can even do this in the bath or shower. Briefly reflect on your interactions today.

Are you holding on to any anger, hatred, or frustration toward someone?

You may find it helpful to do a body scan as described earlier in this chapter. A body scan can be a great tool to uncover any anger, hatred, frustration, or depleting emotion that may present underneath the surface of your awareness.

Is there anyone you need to forgive today?

Replay the events of the day. Is there anyone that you need to forgive (including yourself)? Forgive them, let them go, and set them free. In doing so, you are now free. I like to give the person, situation, and all my thoughts and feelings about it to God and then send the person love and well wishes. It's a powerful act of healing. Forgiveness is about your freedom. It's not about forgetting or accepting that some horrible thing that was said or done was okay. It's about being free from the emotional stranglehold of the person and situation so that you can return to peace, happiness, and wellness within yourself.

Is there anyone that you need to apologize to?

Did you do or say anything today that caused another person pain or harm (intentionally or unintentionally)?

If you feel you need to make amends with someone and apologize, make a note to do it tomorrow and be sure to follow through. You will feel lighter, more free, and likely sleep much better.

This act of taking an evening forgiveness inventory helps to keep things from building up. All the little frustrations and annoyances combined with the big hurts and pains add up if left unchecked, create a radical amount of disharmony in the body and are an immense energy drain on your system. This practice is powerful when practiced with consistency! Forgiveness is an act of radical self-love and a portal back to peace, freedom, and well-being.

Pay Attention to Your Emotional Health

My hope is that by the end of this chapter you will understand the important role emotions play in overall health and the quality of your everyday existence. Learning to become more emotionally intelligent, emotionally resilient in the face of stress, and healing emotional wounds are key considerations when it comes to overcoming chronic health issues and living your best life. Emotions unite mind and body and are critical to address and be aware of when it comes to creating harmony and healing in the body.

Activating core emotions of the heart such as love, gratitude, and care and creating a state of heart coherence as much as possible helps to charge your inner battery, helps improve your resilience to stressful situations, and launches you into a positive thinking and feeling state. This is the state of being that is most conducive to healing and co-creation with the Divine. Engaging the superpowers and daily practices of gratitude and forgiveness are key tools to experiencing more joy, peace, healing, and freedom in your life.

Be sure to make your emotional health and intelligence a priority as you navigate your healing journey! Below you will find a list of some tools and techniques that I have found helpful for myself and my clients in addressing and improving overall emotional health/intelligence, processing emotions, and/or healing emotional wounds.

Tools and Techniques for your Emotions Tool Kit

- HeartMath Tools and Technologies
- Movement:
  - Dancing – I specifically love Gabrielle Roth's 5Rhythms Dance, which can be therapeutic on many different levels
  - Yoga
  - Running/Walking/Hiking
  - Bike riding
  - Any type of exercise you enjoy
- Body/Energy Work
  - Massage
  - Physical therapy
  - Chiropractic adjustments
  - Hugs/physical touch
  - Reiki
  - Acupuncture
  - Craniosacral therapy
  - Breath work/Breathing exercises
- Meditation
- Journaling
- Music and Sound Healing
- Counseling
- Psychotherapy
- Hypnotherapy
- Recall Healing
- Talking to a trusted friend
- Personal Growth Seminars/Coursework
- Crying
- Spending time in nature
- EFT –Emotional Freedom Technique, also known as tapping, is a non-invasive, simple, self-healing practice that involves using your fingers to tap on specific meridian points of the body while

you talk through emotional upsets. It is an excellent, effective, and easily accessible tool to begin releasing negative or depleting emotions.

- Essential oils – Essential oils are the life blood or essence of the plant and contain the plant's immune and protective properties. The essential oil of a plant often contains a very high frequency or vibration, much higher than the human body, and by utilizing it properly through inhalation or topical or internal application you can improve whole-body health by raising the body's vibration. Essential oils also contain numerous healing properties, such as anti-microbial and anti-inflammatory benefits, that can benefit the healing of the physical body (quality is key!). Various essential oils such as bergamot, orange, vetiver, and lavender can help reduce stress and anxiety and can be very effective and powerful emotional healers.

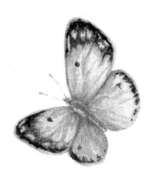

Chapter 7:

Essential #5 –
Live to Thrive: Key Lifestyle Factors

"My mission in life is not merely to survive, but to thrive; and to do
so with some passion, some compassion, some humor, and some style."
– Maya Angelou

Trust me, I know sometimes you may feel like you don't want to get out of bed in the morning and you feel overwhelmed and helpless to change your life situation. Perhaps you're stuck in survival mode and the idea of "thriving" seems like a long shot. I get it. But, in this chapter I will share some simple lifestyle "hacks" that you can implement or address that can get you feeling better and begin to create daily habits to improve your health.

You will notice that many of these lifestyle factors mentioned are quite simple and not rocket science. However, they can pack a huge punch in terms of making a big difference in your health and well-being. Be sure not to overlook them. Go through the topics mentioned in this chapter and take inventory of your life as it is now. Are you doing these things? If so, can you improve in any way? Start with one and fully implement it and then move on to the next!

Sleep

Getting quality and adequate sleep is *crucial* to your body's ability to heal and essential to you feeling well on a day-to-day basis. I know it may seem trivial, but please do *not* underestimate the importance of catching your z's! Lack of sleep can be a common cause of chronic stress (which depletes the immune system and is an underlying factor in all disease) and can negatively impact your mood, make you feel fatigued during the day, promote weight gain, increase your overall risk of chronic disease and impede your healing efforts.[20] Repeated sleep deprivation has been associated with an increased risk for chronic illnesses, such as obesity, type 2 diabetes, cardiovascular disease, hypertension, and mood disorders such as anxiety and depression.[21] No matter what illness you are dealing with, sleep is something you want to make sure that you optimize. Here's how.

1 – Aim for seven to nine hours of sleep in the prime-time window

There's a lot going on while you are sleeping and it is the prime time for your body to *heal*, detoxify, rest, and repair. To take maximum advantage of your body's innate healing abilities it's vitally important that you go to bed by 10:00 p.m. and get seven to nine hours of quality sleep. Between 10 p.m. – 12 a.m. is when your body does some serious healing work and is the time when your immune cells perform the much-needed work of ridding the body of harmful toxins (e.g., viruses, bacteria, and cancer cells). Make sure to take advantage of this! I tell my clients that this is one of those "non-negotiables" if you are healing from any chronic illness or you are just consistently feeling unwell.

Other perks from getting adequate sleep include: improvement in mental clarity and memory so that you can make the best decisions about your health on a daily basis, decreased inflammation, improved mood (which is more conducive to enjoying life), and an overall boost in energy levels. Who doesn't want all that?

2 – Set Yourself Up for Success

Besides getting to sleep by 10 p.m., here are some key things you can do to set yourself up for a good night's sleep:

- ***Avoid electronics before bed***

Shut down *all* electronic devices at *least* thirty minutes before bed. This means avoid checking email, responding to text messages, and scrolling through social media. Not only do these activities have the potential to trigger racing thoughts, but the blue light emitted from electronic devices suppresses melatonin, a key hormone that controls your sleep and wake cycles. The blue light triggers your brain to stay awake even if you feel tired. I recommend and have a pair of blue-light blocking glasses that I wear after sunset that helps relax my eyes and improves my ability to sleep. These are worth checking out, especially if sleep is an issue for you!

- ***Create a sleeping sanctuary***

Make your bedroom into a sanctuary that is an inviting place for you to rest, sleep, cuddle, and make love only. This means avoid working on your computer in bed or bringing any other work or electronic devices into your sleeping environment. Keep your bedroom a "work-free" zone. I recommend removing all electronic devices from your bedroom, including cell phones, televisions, and alarm clocks. These devices emit electromagnetic frequencies and can cause sleep disturbances and insomnia and have been linked to multiple adverse health effects including headaches, depression, anxiety and fatigue, to name a few.[22]

Create a sleep space that is calming – remove the clutter and decorate it in such a way that it makes you feel relaxed when you are in there. I recommend diffusing high quality essentials at night to help induce relaxation. Single essentials such as lavender, vetiver, chamomile, ylang ylang, and frankincense or a combination of relaxing oils can be extremely effective at helping you get a good night's sleep.

Sleep quality is typically improved in a space that is cool and pitch black. As mentioned, lights on at night while you are sleeping can trigger the brain to stay awake. I highly recommend investing in blackout curtains to block any light streaming through your windows – trust me, this can make a huge difference. Remove or cover any other small lights in the room emanating from various devices.

- ***Relax and unwind at least thirty minutes before bed***

So often, we bombard ourselves with information from the television or internet, or work up until bedtime, and then our minds are going a zillion miles an hour and it's tough to fall asleep. I recommend shutting the electronics off thirty minutes before you want to be asleep – so 9:30 would be a good time. In this window, really focus on relaxing and unwinding and consider choosing one or several of the following suggestions:

- Read something positive and relaxing
- Take a bath with high-quality essential oils and/or Epsom salt
- Do some deep breathing
- Practice heart coherence (see Chapter 6)
- Do gentle stretching
- Meditate or pray
- Write in a journal
- Brain dump – If your mind is racing from a stressful day, try doing a "brain dump." Instead of going to bed with an endless to-do list weighing on you, grab a pen and paper and "dump" it all out.
- Give yourself a foot massage (or trade with your partner)
- Drink a calming tea – best not to do this too close to bed to avoid having to get up in the night to pee

Movement

Movement is an important component to include in your daily routine – whether you are healing from a chronic illness or you just want to feel good as you age. Notice how I didn't use the word "exercise." I find that some women have an aversion to that word and it means a lot of different things to a lot of different people. When it comes to healing your body and your life it's important to incorporate some type of movement, so I will provide some recommendations and guidelines here. As with all recommendations in this book, you must always listen to your body and feel into what is best for you and/or seek out a qualified health practitioner to get individualized guidance. Depending on your functional ability and energy levels, incorporating movement in your life could look like anything from a five to ten minute walk every day or doing gentle stretching in your bed to doing light resistance training.

Permission to Slow Down

Strenuous exercise and long duration "cardio" exercise is not ideal or beneficial to those deep in their healing journey. This type of movement or exercise places further stress on the body, drains the resources your body needs to heal, and depletes the immune system. Being an athlete my whole life, training hard and hitting the gym most days was the norm for me. When I was incredibly sick and experiencing immense fatigue, I could hardly walk up the stairs of our condominium. Yet, I still felt guilty that I wasn't working out. I very much had my identity and worth wrapped up in being an athlete and felt awful about myself and extremely critical when I could no longer do the things I used to do. And when I did have good days I would completely ruin my progress by "overdoing it" and it would knock me back down (sometimes worse) than I was before. I finally figured out that exercise *had* to look different for me at that time, and that was okay. The mental stress of feeling guilty or inadequate or the physical stress of pushing myself to lift weights was not conducive to my healing.

Check in with yourself. Are you overdoing it? Are you placing ridiculously high expectations on yourself that lead to angst, guilt, and shame?

None of this is conducive to your healing. Really begin to learn how to tune into your body and meet yourself where you are today (not yesterday or three years ago) with love, compassion, and gratitude.

Health Benefits

No matter where you are in your healing journey, some type of movement is important to the healing of your whole being. Movement/exercise helps to improve circulation, detoxify or clear the body and lymphatic system of toxins, boost immune function, enhance your mood, decrease stress, and help you to maintain your functional ability, and can also help to decrease pain.

We know that consistent physical activity reduces the risk of many chronic diseases, such as cardiovascular disease, diabetes, cancer, hypertension, obesity, depression, and osteoporosis.[23] And we also know that being sedentary substantially increases your risk of chronic disease, especially those that sit or are sedentary for more than six to eight hours a day. Chronic sitting increases risk for developing chronic disease conditions such as heart disease and Type II diabetes,[24] and is associated with the development of chronic and acute pain and a decline in functional mobility over time. All this is to say, consistent movement that is in alignment with your current functional ability and health, and avoiding prolonged sitting if possible is important to your healing journey.

Get Moving

If you are currently not doing any movement at all (and you are able), start with a five to ten-minute walk in the morning and evening. Although super simple, walking outside in nature while getting some sunshine is a powerful healing tonic for body, mind, and spirit. Sometimes, I like to take my shoes off and walk barefoot around the lake by our house. The energy from the earth is incredibly grounding and healing and I highly recommend it. If you aren't able to walk, there are plenty of exercises that can be performed in a chair or lying down. Work with a physical therapist or qualified trainer to come up with a routine that works for you.

Depending on where you are in your healing journey, here are some lower impact movement/exercise modalities that may be good options for you. I recommend finding one or several methods of movement that you enjoy! You are much more likely to be consistent if you enjoy it.

Gentle Healing Movement Practices
- Walking
- Water walking/jogging – Water walking involves using a flotation belt around your mid-section and allows you to walk/jog in the water without any impact on your joints.
- Swimming
- Hiking
- Bike Riding
- Rebounding – Rebounding involves jumping up and down on a mini trampoline or rebounder and is a great way to get exercise and cleanse the lymphatic system!
- Dancing – (i.e. 5Rhythms, Qoya, ecstatic dance)
- Yoga (i.e. Yin, Chair, Kundalini)
- Tai Chi
- Qigong
- Functional body weight exercises (i.e. – squats, planks, lunges)
- Light resistance exercise using resistance bands or light weights

Sunshine and Nature
I love how intuitive our little Goldendoodle, Maya, is. Your dog, if you have one, may do this too. Frequently I find her sunning herself on the porch or inside next to the window. She instinctively knows it's good for her body and you can tell she's enjoying it. Nothing beats feeling a bit

chilled and then spending a few moments basking in the sunshine and letting the sun warm and nourish you from the outside in.

Sunshine is another powerful, yet simple and often overlooked piece of the healing puzzle. The health benefits of sunshine include boosting immunity, improving sleep, elevating mood, decreasing inflammation, improving bone health, and reducing risk of certain cancers, cardiovascular disease, autoimmune conditions, and neurodegenerative disease.[25]

The most important benefit of sun exposure is that it provides your body with Vitamin D, which is a critical hormone that is involved in numerous bodily functions and metabolic processes. At least half of the world (or more) is deficient in vitamin D, which may be due to the fear around skin cancer and sun exposure. People have become afraid to get *any* sun exposure, so they lather on sunscreen which, unfortunately, often contains carcinogenic chemicals and prevents them from receiving the much-needed vitamin D that helps prevent cancer and other chronic diseases. Low levels of vitamin D have been linked to many disease conditions including, cancer, Alzheimer's, Type II diabetes, asthma, cardiovascular disease, osteoporosis, and autoimmune diseases.[26]

Getting Sunshine

Make getting *healthy* sun exposure on your bare skin a priority; however, it is very important that you *avoid* getting burned. Try to get between at least ten minutes to approximately thirty minutes of sunshine a day (again, without getting burned). Don't use sunscreen during this time period, as that would prevent you from getting the UV rays you need to make vitamin D. The appropriate amount of sun exposure varies based on the individual, geographic location, skin color, and weight. Darker skinned people require more sun exposure to get the same amount of vitamin D as it does for lighter-skinned folks. If you are out in the sun all day, get a small dose of sunshine and then protect yourself with shade, clothing, or a toxin-free sunscreen.

Let Nature Nurture You

Our modern society has lost touch with nature and the impact is devastating – individually and collectively. We spend so much time in front of electronic devices and in the hustle and bustle of living that we have become disconnected from Mother Earth – the very source of what sustains our life. We are wise to glean wisdom from our ancestors and indigenous tribes still existing that live in harmony with and are very connected to nature, revering Her for Her physical and spiritual sustenance She provides. We forget how Mother Nature supports us and provides for our needs without asking anything in return. The plants of the earth nourish us, heal us, provide the oxygen we require to live, teach us, clothe us, and provide shelter. From the intricacy and vibrant colors of all the many unique and different flowers, to an exquisite and colorful sunset, to the greatness of a whale, to the delicate perfection of a butterfly wing, to our own unique thumbprint – we are reminded of the complexity, creativity, and imagination of the Creator and the interconnectedness of all living things.

Unfortunately, the majority of our modern culture has lost its reverence for the Earth, our sense of what is sacred, and our knowingness of who we are as spiritual beings – it is reflected in the destroying of our planet, the violence, the epidemic disease, and the disconnectedness we feel that no amount of money, fame, or power can remedy. As we restore our sense of wholeness, we realize that we are intimately connected to earth and all of Life. Being in nature helps us to remember who we are and helps us reorient to our truest and highest Self. Taking the time in nature – walking, hiking, swimming, camping, or playing – helps us get away from the busyness of life, put things into perspective, nourish our soul and reminds us to let go of the small and insignificant stuff that doesn't serve us.

There is a magic and a powerful healing energy that exists when you spend time consistently in nature. We've talked about the healing power of sunshine, but the air, the wind, the water, and earth can all help you restore balance and harmony to your being. Have you ever noticed you felt really good after walking on the beach all day? I always feel significantly better when I spend the day barefoot at the beach and have since taken up walking barefoot around the lake where I live. Although I'm sure it's a combination of many of the elements – sunshine, saltwater, and fresh air – as well as feeling more relaxed just being in nature, there's actually some profound healing power that comes from being barefoot on the earth.

Earthing, as it is called, involves "coupling" or making actual contact with your bare feet or body to the earth, which infuses your body with negative-charged free electrons that are abundant on the Earth's surface. The body equalizes to the same electrical energy level of the Earth. Some healing benefits that have been associated with earthing are: decreased inflammation, decreased pain, improved sleep, increased energy, accelerated healing, and reduced stress. (Note: There are also earthing devices (sheets, mats to sit on) that allow you to reap the same benefits while indoors).[27]

Did you know that spending time in nature decreases stress, increases relaxation, and can actually improve immunity? Amazing, right?! Have you heard of "forest bathing"? Forest bathing involves hanging out and walking in the forest for a few days – like a weekend camping trip. Some researchers studied the effects of forest bathing on our health. They found that just being immersed in the forest increased immune function and improved stress levels. They even suggested that "forest bathing trips may have a preventive effect on cancer generation and development." How awesome are trees?! Trees even express essential oil compounds that you breathe in while in nature that have a relaxing effect on the body and help you to decrease stress. [28] I highly recommend spending some time in nature every single day.

Here are some ideas to get more of nature's medicine in your life:

- Go outside at your lunch break at work. Take your shoes off and let your feet be in the grass while you sit at a picnic table.

- Get up a little earlier and spend some time sipping tea on your back patio and watch the birds.
- Come home at the end of the day and go for a walk in nature instead of watching TV.
- Work out outside with bare feet instead of in the gym (as long as the weather is appropriate).
- Get some house plants!
- Plan vacations around visiting beautiful places in nature.
- Find a place close to you that has a hiking trail and go hike.
- Have a picnic on the ground with someone you love.
- Plant some flowers or herbs in your backyard.
- Choose to live close to nature if you are able.
- Hug a tree! Yes. Seriously.

Brainstorm ways you can let nature nurture you daily. Be consistent with your daily dose of nature for a couple weeks and see what you notice!

Play

I used to believe that play was a luxury for us adults – something that people who had money and free time could do. Or I thought playing could happen if you had kids, of course, but I didn't have any kids so playing was something I did not do with any regularity. I often felt guilty or stressed about the idea of playing and having fun and thought I was wasting precious time that could and should be used being "productive." I think most of the adult population is the same way. We think one day when we have more time, accomplish "the thing" and make the money, we can take more vacations and spend more time playing and doing the things that we enjoy. We are ruled by pressure to do, to be, and to have. When we live in such a way where we are constantly on the go, do-do-do, no time to rest, push harder – without leaving time for rest or fun – it is a recipe for stress, illness, apathy and depression. And yet we have an entire culture that operates under the belief that this is the way we have to do things. But, we can actually choose differently.

What we don't realize is that play actually helps us achieve our dreams with more ease and joy. When we follow our joy, we are following the path to our own unique purpose and the dreams of our heart. Shifting our mindset from pressure to pleasure can open up a whole new experience of life on this planet – one of more joy, peace, and well-being. Play helps us do this. Play is crucial for creativity, helps us to relax, improves our ability to imagine, boosts mood, enhances connection with nature and each other, and improves learning. It helps lift our moods and supercharges our creative juices, helping us to live from that place of creation mode versus being stuck in stress and survival mode. Play actually helps us achieve all the things we are striving to attain in a much healthier and more joyful way. Who doesn't want that?

Take the time every day to play a little bit or even a lot! Having a dog or a pet is super helpful to remind you to play and rest. We need both to heal and thrive! We all have different things that are fun to us. Do what is fun and uplifting to you – without stress, without guilt, and feel good knowing you are doing something to help you heal, be more creative, and even be *more* productive while you are working. What would living look like if you let ease and pleasure guide you versus putting so much pressure on yourself? So, maybe you have quite a bit of work to do on the computer today. What if you took a couple breaks today and cranked the music up and danced around your home office for ten minutes and took another break and played with dog in the backyard? How might you feel different at the end of your work day? Brainstorm ways you can infuse more play into your every day.

Laughter

How long has it been since you had a good belly-laugh or laughed so hard you were crying? Remember how amazing that feels? Laughter is some of the best medicine – not only for your soul, but your body too. I recall hearing about a man during the cancer part of my healing journey, Dr. Norman Cousins, who claimed it was lots of laughter and vitamins that healed him of ankylosing spondylitis – a painful and degenerative condition of the spine that has no cure. He watched hours and hours of funny movies and reported that ten minutes of belly laughter helped him to sleep pain-free for two hours when even morphine couldn't. He completely recovered from his "incurable" condition and went on to write a book about his extraordinary experience in his book called *Anatomy of Illness*.

Inspired by Cousins, I made a decision during my healing journey, especially after my surgery, to watch as many funny, uplifting movies (and some comedy shows too) as I could. I remember how good it felt to laugh! It's so easy to get sucked into the doom and gloom when you feel sick. Life begins to feel heavy, scary, overwhelming and way too serious. Use laughter, as well as gratitude, to bounce back to joy! Thinking and feeling beyond your current circumstances and in alignment with your vision of your health helps you to create that which you desire. It's in the positive uplifting emotions of love, appreciation, compassion, and care that help you achieve harmony and healing in your life. Adding laughter brings joy to your heart and creates an internal environment conducive to healing. There has even been some research on the topic of laughter and its associated health benefits, so why not make it a point to laugh daily? It's free and there are no negative side effects (unless you call laughing so hard you pee yourself one!).

Laughter may help improve overall well-being by:[29]
- Reducing stress (extremely important!)
- Relaxing the muscles in the body
- Triggering natural release of endorphins and relieving pain
- Enhancing oxygen uptake
- Increasing positive emotions and attitude
- Improving sleep
- Enhancing quality of life
- Enhancing connection and social bonds
- Balancing blood pressure
- Improving memory and learning

Reduce Toxin Exposure

Accumulated toxicity in the body is one of the key culprits when it comes to chronic illness. Reducing your daily exposure to toxicity in your environment, as well as clearing toxins from the body, is an extremely important component to restoring your health. Toxins are essentially poisons or substances that are capable of producing illness or death. News-flash – we, unfortunately, live in a toxic soup and are exposed to over five hundred toxic substances on a *daily* basis.[30]

There are thousands of chemicals added to our food supply, used in food processing, and lurking in our personal care products and cleaning supplies. Many of these noxious chemicals don't have to be listed on the label *and* most have *not* been thoroughly tested on how they affect human biology. Before we even take our first breath on this planet, we likely have toxic chemicals in our bodies passed to us from our parents. Research reveals that an average of two hundred+ toxic chemicals were found in the cord blood of newborn babies, not to mention that the average American carries a "body burden" of seven hundred synthetic chemicals![31]

The chemicals and toxic substances we are exposed to on a daily basis *accumulate* and negatively impact the body by weakening the immune system, creating hormone imbalances, causing digestive distress, interfering with the body's ability to detoxify, accelerating aging, and increasing risk of developing chronic disease conditions such as cancer, neurological conditions, autoimmune disease, cardiovascular disease, depression, allergies, asthma, and infertility.[32] Our daily exposure and accumulation of toxins in our food, water, air, homes, and environment is a huge reason why chronic illness is so rampant.

According to Dr. Pizzorno, founder of Bastyr University and author of *The Toxin Solution*, "Toxins are now the *primary* cause of chronic disease. They are driving much of what we see as clinicians. We need to reckon with the fact that our population is incredibly sick, and toxins are a major driver."

Bottom line – decreasing exposure to the daily bombardment of toxins is a *critical* component in recovering from chronic illness. The accumulation of toxins in your body is likely a big reason why your body may be having a hard time healing. I share these statistics with you not to make you feel afraid of your environment, because living in fear is just as problematic as the toxic chemical. My intention is to help you become aware so that you can make empowered choices regarding what you eat, drink, and breathe, and how you live.

Not only is it important to do specific detoxification work to clear your body of years of accumulated toxins, but it's important to remove and clear toxins from your home and environment in order to decrease daily exposure. Toxins are blocking factors to your healing. Period.

Here is an overview of some of the toxins that you may find in your environment:

- Food: pesticides, herbicides, fungicides, heavy metals, hormones, GMOs (genetically modified organisms), and other food additives
- Water: chemicals (aluminum, chlorine, chloramines, etc.), heavy metals, pathogens, pharmaceutical residue, and more
- Industrial Chemicals: chemicals from industrial manufacturing and runoff, chemical off-gassing from paints and dyes, manufactured furniture, car interior fabrics, plastics, and many other modern accommodations
- Chemicals in personal care/body care products
- Chemicals in household cleaners and lawn maintenance
- Electromagnetic fields (EMFs)
- Drug use (including OTC/prescription and illegal)
- Alcohol and cigarettes

In this chapter, we will focus on what we can do in our own homes and environments to reduce or eliminate toxin exposure. Next chapter, we will discuss toxins in food and water. As for alcohol, illegal drug use, and cigarettes, I recommend avoiding them entirely. When it comes to OTC/prescription drugs, you will have to use discernment and discuss this with your doctor; however, I do recommend learning about natural alternatives. There are many incredible tools like herbs, essential oils, and homeopathic remedies that are very effective when it comes to addressing things like colds, flu, rashes, etc. without negative side effects. There is always going to be a certain level of industrial chemicals and toxin exposure that we don't have control over, so for our purposes we will focus on what we do have control over!

Household Toxins

It's likely that you spend a significant amount of time in your home and you want it to be a space conducive to deep healing and rejuvenation. To accomplish this, you want to make sure you ditch or swap out toxic items that may be sabotaging your healing efforts. These chemicals may be lurking in your cleaning products, kitchen cookware, food/water containers, and air. I will discuss these below. These upgrades may require a financial commitment, so make them at your own pace, but know they are totally worth the investment and will be very important in your long-term health.

All Cleaning Products

I recommend ditching all industrial chemical cleaning products and replace them with natural, non-toxic cleaning products made with essential oils or natural, simple ingredients. There are safe, non-toxic cleaner options for everything from all-purpose cleaners, to dish soap, and laundry detergent. You can go to the Environmental Working Group's website, which is an extraordinary tool and database, to find the best non-toxic cleaners for your home, or you can also consider making DIY (Do It Yourself) natural cleaners using high quality essential oils (you can find many recipes online). Take an inventory of what you have and if it contains a ton of chemicals and has a pungent chemical smell, replace it with a safer, natural option.

Kitchen Cookware

Get rid of all Teflon nonstick cookware. Although these types of pots and pans make cooking super quick and easy, it is not worth the toxic chemicals that leach into your food and air and wreak havoc on your body! Teflon is made of a chemical known as PFOA and has been shown to cause cancer, liver damage, growth defects, immune system compromise, and death in lab animals. It is also advisable to avoid aluminum cookware. Aluminum may have detrimental effects on the nervous system and may be linked to neurological conditions such as Alzheimer's, autism spectrum disorders, and multiple sclerosis.[33]

- Avoid:
  - Teflon nonstick cookware
  - Aluminum cookware
- Switch to:
  - Ceramic
  - Cast iron ceramic-coated cookware
  - Glass
  - Stainless steel

Food/Water Storage

Avoid storing food and water in plastic. Many plastics and storage containers made of plastic contain the toxic chemicals BPA and phthalates. Steer clear of these! Both of these chemicals are hormone disruptors and have been linked to cancer, heart disease, brain and behavior changes, and dysfunction of the reproductive system.[34]

These harmful chemicals are known to leach into the food and water from the containers that store them. Also avoid using Styrofoam, especially heating it, which may cause DNA damage, reduce glutathione levels, and has estrogenic properties.[35]

- Avoid:
  - Plastic food storage containers
  - Plastic wrap

        ▫   Storing food in plastic Ziploc bags
        ▫   All plastic water bottles
        ▫   Plastic utensils and cups
        ▫   Styrofoam cups and plates

- Switch to:
  - ▫   Glass food storage containers
  - ▫   Glass mason jars for food/beverage storage
  - ▫   Glass water bottles

Airborne Toxins

Most humans spend the majority of time indoors. It is estimated that our indoor air pollution is two to five times more polluted than our outdoor air.[36] Can you believe that?! Be aware of items that off-gas or produce chemicals into the air that you may be breathing in consistently inside your home.

Here are some key items that can contain compounds that are harmful when inhaled:

- Household cleaners
- Furniture polish
- Paint thinner
- Paints
- Air fresheners/fragrances
- Artificial candles
- Pesticides
- Dry cleaning chemicals
- Nonstick cookware
- Mold
- New building materials – furniture, carpet

Get rid of synthetic scents that fill the air with chemicals, such as air fresheners and artificial candles, and replace them with natural options.

There are naturally made, non-toxic candles available for purchase and diffusing high quality essential oils not only makes the room smell good, but cleans the air and has added mood and health benefits. Many high-quality essential oils are naturally anti-viral and anti-bacterial and can clear these things from the air as well. Do your best to remove things that off-gas chemicals into the air and keep them out of your home environment. I highly recommend using natural solutions for bug and pest control versus spraying your home with pesticides.

Personal Care Products

Women use a smorgasbord of skincare and beauty products on a daily basis – from mascara, to lotion, hairspray, lipstick, and perfume. You won't believe it, but the average woman exposes herself to 515 synthetic chemicals in her daily grooming and make-up routine.[37] That's a lot of chemicals! It's important to understand that much of what we put on our skin absorbs into our bloodstreams and into our bodies. Many of these dangerous chemicals can be found in cosmetics. It is estimated that 65% of women's cosmetics contain potentially carcinogenic ingredients.[38]

The truth is that we lather, spritz, and spray concoctions of chemicals that are known neurotoxins, hormone disruptors, carcinogens, and known to damage or disrupt various organs and system of the body. If you're like me, I used to never look at ingredients on anything. But once I started learning about all the junk in our food supply, I began researching the ingredients in my personal care products too. I found that so many of the ingredients were toxic and had dangerous side effects. I was infuriated and felt betrayed! One would think and hope that if the deodorant I'm slathering on my armpits every day contains toxic chemicals then they wouldn't put it on the market. Unfortunately, that's not the case. As mentioned, there is not much regulation on these products. Our society is very focused on beauty and aesthetics and these large make-up and personal care product companies make *a lot* of money when we buy their stuff. It's important that we become more aware, begin to make different choices, and demand cleaner, healthier products if we want to get well and stay well.

When we add these chemicals, from personal care products to the chemicals found in food, water, air, and in our cleaners ... it adds up pretty fast. The body is well-equipped with an incredible detoxification system; however, it often cannot keep up at the rate at which we expose our bodies to toxic chemicals. The accumulated toxicity in your body's chemistry (and consciousness) is what leads to disease.

Personal Care Product Makeover

Okay ... it's time to ditch the toxic make-up and lotions. In general, you want to look for skin, body, hair, and oral care products that contain simple, organic, and natural ingredients. The simpler the better. The Environmental Working Group (EWG) also has an incredibly informative and comprehensive database of various cosmetic and personal care products. It rates many of the products on the market on how toxic they are and lists their ingredients and any negative health effects. It's an invaluable resource, so use it to help you find natural, clean products.

Here's a great way to makeover your personal care products using the EWG database:

1. Do an inventory of your current personal care products. Check your toiletries, shower items, make-up bag, and don't forget your feminine hygiene products! Use the list below for reference.
2. Cross check your products with the EWG website.
3. Only keep those that are in the "low" toxicity range.
4. If they are in the medium to high range – ditch them.
5. Replace them with products in the "low" toxicity range.

Here's a list of the common personal care products to address:
- make-up

- lotions
- body soap
- deodorant
- hair dyes
- hair sprays and gels
- toothpaste
- shampoos/conditioners
- hand soap
  - Avoid antibacterial hand soap, which contains triclosan, a substance that interferes with hormone function and is a potential culprit in antibiotic resistance, which is a growing health concern.[39]
- feminine hygiene products
  - Pads and tampons contain toxic chemicals such as BPA, phthalates, and chlorine bleach, so swap them out for 100% organic cotton options.

Another great option is to make your own lotions, deodorant, and toothpowders. This is a great way to assure you have the highest-quality ingredients. There are many amazing DIY blogs and websites out there that teach you how to make organic, high-quality personal care products. If you are dealing with low energy or have a lot on your plate, it may be easiest just to buy them. Keep in mind, some of the smaller companies may not be on the EWG website, but still may be great options. I often find great skincare at farmer's markets made organically, in small batches, with high-quality ingredients that I can pronounce and without chemicals. You can also look for natural, organic products with simple ingredients at many natural health food stores. However, keep in mind, just because it says "natural" doesn't necessarily mean it's free of harmful ingredients. You may not be able to afford to ditch everything at once and get new stuff. Pick one thing at a time and gradually replace them all. Your body will thank you!

Electromagnetic Fields (EMFs)

Electromagnetic fields are a pervasive environmental toxin that you are exposed to every day that could be sabotaging your health (and is one major downside when it comes to modern technology). Dr. Milham, author of *Dirty Electricity*, points to the recent proliferation of EMFs from various sources as a key factor in increasing rates of chronic diseases such as cancer, cardiovascular disease, and diabetes. Even the WHO's International Agency for Research on Cancer (IARC) declared cell phones and Wi-Fi to be "Group 2B Possible Carcinogens," or possible cancer-causing agents.[40] EMF exposure has also been linked to brain and nervous system disorders such as autism, depression, Alzheimer's, insomnia, depressed immunity, hormone imbalances, sleep disturbances, fatigue, headaches, and more.[41]

EMF exposure comes from different sources in your environment and is cumulative in its effects on your body. One of the main sources of EMF exposure is your cell phone (which most humans on the planet use every day). Other sources include wireless phones, computers, Wi-Fi, and cell phone towers. Just because you can't see EMFs or directly feel them doesn't mean they are aren't impacting your body. EMFs are invisible and can move through walls and solid substances such as brick and wood. It's important to do your best to decrease your exposure to EMFs as much as possible.

Here are a few practical ways you can decrease your EMF exposure:
- Do not place your cell phone directly to your ear when talking. Use your speaker phone or earbuds instead.
- Do not carry your cell phone in your pocket or on your body. Ladies, please don't put your cell phone in your bra!
- Keep your cell phone six feet or more away from your body when not in use.
- Avoid using your cell phone when the signal strength is low.
- Put your phone on airplane mode when you aren't using it.

- Minimize or avoid using your cell phone while driving. Radiation levels are higher when you are moving than when you are stationary.
- Replace Wi-Fi installation with wired internet.
- Turn off all electronic devices at night, including your Wi-Fi router if possible.
- Avoid using your laptop on your lap.
- Avoid using your laptop on the main power supply.
- Consider investing in quality EMF protection.
  - Dr. Véronique Desaulniers, holistic breast cancer doctor, recommends products from GIA Wellness as the best technology she's found for optimal protection. I have a pendant from GIA Wellness that I wear while on my laptop to protect me while I am on the computer.

Simple Yet Foundational

Getting adequate sleep and sunshine, moving your body, spending time in nature, reducing toxin exposure, and playing and laughing on a daily basis are all key things that are extremely important for you in your healing journey. Many of these things not only increase your overall well-being and balance your body, mind, heart and soul, but also bring more peace, joy, and connection to your life.

These lifestyle factors are the foundation to living a healthy and happy life! Take the time and consideration to see where you could add or improve upon these essential elements. Master these basics and refrain from skipping over them due to simplicity. Don't try to take on everything at once. Pick one thing at a time, get familiar with it, and implement or upgrade it until it's part of your daily life, then move on to the next thing! I know you can do it, and trust me, you'll be happy you did!

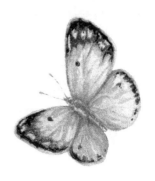

Chapter 8:

Essential #6 –
Eat, Drink, Detox

"Let food be thy medicine and medicine be thy food."
– Hippocrates

Eat

What the heck am I supposed to eat? It's likely that you've bumped up against this question one too many times for your liking during your quest to get well. It can be overwhelming and maddening to figure out what foods to eat, what not to eat, or what diet to follow. Food plays a foundational role when it comes to getting and staying well. During just the cancer part of my journey I worked with five different (highly trained, highly sought-after) practitioners and they all had different takes on what I should be eating – from a modified ketogenic diet, to vegan, to large amounts of juicing and fasting, eat fish, don't eat fish because of the polluted oceans – ahhhh. It was confusing – and I was a health practitioner who had been studying nutrition and natural healing for years, and I was still confused!

Chronic illness constitutes a wide spectrum of health issues manifesting as a conglomeration of symptoms and labels called "diagnoses" that I don't particularly choose to get wrapped up in. What I'd like to provide is a general starting place and recommendations of foods to avoid that create toxicity in the body and foods that nourish and heal (generally speaking). It's important to understand that every person is different and what's uber healthy for one person can be inflammatory for another. For example, most all diets agree vegetables and fruits are healthy. Tomatoes fall in that category. When I eat tomatoes and foods in the *nightshade family I immediately get sores in my mouth and congestion in my head and sinuses. Tomatoes are a no-go for me, but they have many healing properties and can be super-healthy for other people. Be mindful of this as you tune-into which foods are best for you.

(*Note: Nightshades are a group of vegetables in the Solanaceae family and include tomatoes, bell peppers, white potatoes, eggplants, tomatillos, peppers, etc. Look online for a complete list. These vegetables contain glycoalkaloids that can cause digestive upset and inflammation in some people. If you are dealing with an autoimmune condition, arthritis, or a digestive disorder like leaky gut, Celiac Disease, or Irritable Bowel Syndrome (IBS), you may consider removing nightshades from your diet to see how that makes you feel.)[42]

We've been talking a lot about following your intuition and listening to your heart to help you navigate your healing path. Use your intuition and listen to your body when it comes to food as well; it can be a very helpful guide. The key is slowing down long enough to listen. I kid you not, when I was in graduate school we would all go to Buffalo Wild Wings to let off some steam and I would polish off a basket of hot wings (yep ... nightshade-smothered wings). Afterwards, as early as the drive home, my stomach would be in knots and I would be doubled over in pain. But, did it deter me from going back to chow down more? Nope. Sadly, I was completely disconnected from listening to my body. I shrugged off the stabbing stomach pain, popped some antacid, moved on to studying or the next to-do in my day, and then found myself back at the hot wing joint scarfing down more hot wings a couple weeks later. Not that poor food choices were the only culprit, but a few years later I became very ill with obvious gut and immune related symptoms. The moral of the story is pay attention. Your body talks, so be sure to listen!

Food Journal

Consciously create awareness of how the foods you eat make you feel. One excellent tool for this is a food journal. I have all my clients do this for at least three to seven days to help them gain awareness about what they are eating, how often and when they are eating, and how they feel after eating meals. I highly recommend you give this a try. Essentially, all you do is write down what you eat for each meal and snack (including which cooking oils/fats and condiments you use) and track how that food makes you feel afterwards. You may notice things like fatigue, headaches, stomach pain, or low/high energy after you eat a particular meal. If you keep meals very simple, you can begin to single out foods that you may be poorly tolerating.

On the same paper for the day, I also recommend tracking your water intake to keep track of how well you are hydrating yourself. You can also track your bowel movements, which can be a helpful source of information (use a Bristol Stool Chart, which you can find online). You may notice that certain foods give you loose stools or notice undigested food in your stool indicating you aren't breaking down your food well and/or chewing well enough. These can be indications that the foods you are eating may not be good choices for you.

Use the following recommendations as a foundation for your dietary approach along with your intuition, and ideally combined with a trusted practitioner to help you make decisions about what is ideal for you and your particular health challenge. Use this chapter as a starting place and then expand from here to find your sweet spot.

Food as Medicine

Food can be medicine, or it can literally make you sick. In our modern culture we've gotten so off track when it comes to food. The majority of the food we eat is fast and quick. It may be conducive to keeping up in such a faced-paced world, but it's highly processed, chemicalized, and engineered – and happens to be one of the culprits in the chronic disease epidemic. If you want to get and stay well you must *slow down*, simplify, and return to eating food in its most natural, whole, nutrient-dense form and do your best to eliminate toxic and inflammatory foods. Eating this way involves ditching most of the packages, boxes, and cans that are largely devoid of nutrients and often contain harmful ingredients, and choosing to consume foods with the most nutrition and health-promoting, life-giving compounds. While this involves spending a little more time shopping, preparing, and cooking your food, versus stopping through the drive through or popping a frozen dinner in the microwave, the extra time spent is worth its weight in gold when it comes to healing and feeling good.

Foods to Focus on
1) Vegetables and Fruits

A diet rich in vegetables and fruits is an important part of a healing regimen. Mother Nature has provided a cornucopia of colorful vegetables and fruits that are packed with healing compounds and protect against illness. When you take advantage of "eating the rainbow" you benefit from the wide range of available vitamins, minerals, phytonutrients, and healing properties. For example, orange/yellow fruits and vegetables such as oranges and carrots are rich in vitamin C and carotenoids, which are known for supporting the immune system and promoting eye health. Blue and purple fruits and vegetables, such as blueberries and purple cabbage, contain anthocyanins and resveratrol, which are known for their anti-cancer, antioxidant, and anti-aging properties. Fruits and vegetables are also excellent sources of fiber, which promote good bowel health.

<u>Veggies</u>

Most diets can agree and so do I, that vegetables are key. I recommend eating an abundance and variety of veggies. Fill your plate with mostly veggies and remember to include a variety to take advantage of their different healing properties. Make sure to include raw veggies daily in your diet (if you can tolerate them) in order to take advantage of the high levels of bio-available enzymes, which help boost digestion and optimize health. Most people eat the majority of their food cooked, which inevitably destroys some nutrients and enzymes. Get in the habit of eating a big leafy green salad that includes all the colors of the rainbow. For example, add the following to your plate of greens: radishes (red), carrots (orange/yellow), shredded purple cabbage (purple/blue), green apples (white/green). Top with some broccoli sprouts, avocado, ground flax seeds, and a homemade olive oil and apple cider vinegar dressing and you've got a power-packed salad!

I highly recommend including cruciferous vegetables in your diet with consistency (if well tolerated). These veggies in particular are powerhouses of nutrition because they contain a particular phytochemical in abundance: sulforaphane. Sulforaphane has a host of healing properties including helping to protect and eliminate toxins from the body and contains potent anti-cancer and antioxidant properties.[43]

Broccoli, arugula, bok choy, turnips, watercress, cauliflower, radishes, cabbage, Brussels sprouts, and kale are examples of cruciferous vegetables. Broccoli sprouts in particular are loaded with sulforaphane and I highly recommend you include them in your diet. Sprouts of all kinds, including broccoli sprouts, are easy to grow at home, have a ton of nutrients and can be added easily to salads and smoothies.

Here are some ways you can prepare your veggies. Mix it up and use a variety of herbs and spices to keep the flavors interesting!
- raw salads
- hot puréed and chunky soups as well as cold raw soups
- veggie stir-fries

- roasted veggies
- mashes (e.g., cauliflower or sweet potato mash)

Fruits

Fruits are the highest electrically-alkaline foods, as well as excellent brain and nerve foods. They are high in antioxidants and astringent properties, which make them powerful cleansers. It's best to consume fruits alone (not combined with proteins or fats) for optimal digestion and to tap into their cleansing and regenerative properties. Melons especially are best eaten by themselves because they digest so quickly (which takes approximately twenty minutes). When they are eaten with harder to digest foods, it results in fermentation and undigested sugar in the gut, which can be problematic. Melons are easy to digest, and contain a large amount of structured water, making them excellent hydrators and cleansers.[44]

Produce Quality

In order to choose the highest-quality fruits and vegetables, do your best to get organic, which ensures your produce is free of herbicides, pesticides, and GMOs (genetically modified organisms – we will discuss this in detail in the next couple sections). Unfortunately, a strawberry isn't necessarily *just* a strawberry anymore. Even once you decide to eat whole, real food you still have to be concerned with quality to make sure you are eating something that is healing versus toxic to your body. Conventional produce found in our grocery stores contains a wide range of potentially hazardous chemicals. For example, according to tests run by the U.S. Department of Agriculture in 2015 and 2016, strawberries contained an average of 7.8 different pesticides per sample, while the dirtiest samples contained twenty-two pesticides and breakdown products. Some of these chemicals used have been linked to cancer, reproductive and developmental damage, hormone disruption, or neurological issues.[45]

Choose organic if possible or at least shop using the Environmental Working Group's (EWG) Dirty Dozen and Clean 15 guide that can be found online. This list will help you know which fruits and vegetables you should buy organic (these have the most toxins) and which ones you could opt for conventional (these have the lowest levels of toxins). If you are shopping at a farmer's market, be aware that produce from small farmers may not be labeled "organic" because they cannot afford the certification process but may still use organic farming practices. Simply ask if they use herbicides and pesticides in their farming practices.

2) Herbs and Spices

Herbs and spices are powerful and inexpensive natural medicines, so be sure to take advantage by incorporating them into your meals daily. In addition to containing an abundance of healing properties, they provide a radical amount of depth and flavor to your food and help to keep meals from getting boring. Consider adding fresh, chopped herbs to stir-fries and salads, making pestos out of basil and garlic, juicing parsley and ginger in your green juices, and experimenting with a variety of spices in dishes. Herbs such as oregano, thyme, and rosemary are easy to grow in your garden, on your windowsill, or on your balcony. Herbs and spices can be potent anti-inflammatories, boost the immune system, and be a powerful defense against pathogens and disease.

Here's a list of the top seven herbs and spices that I recommend using in your healing regimen to reduce inflammation and boost immunity:

1. cayenne (as long as you aren't sensitive to nightshades)
2. cinnamon
3. cloves
4. garlic
5. ginger
6. rosemary
7. turmeric

3) Nuts and Seeds

Nuts and seeds are great structural foods for strengthening the body and glands and contain vitamins, minerals such as magnesium and selenium, and omega 3 fatty acids (also supportive of bone/joint, heart and brain health). Seek out organic, raw nuts and seeds and avoid fried, candied, or roasted nuts that use unhealthy industrial seed vegetable oils such as soybean or canola. Check your labels.

Nuts and seeds such as macadamia nuts, almonds, walnuts, brazil nuts, pumpkin seeds, sunflower seeds, flax seeds, hempseeds, and chia seeds are some of the healthiest nuts and seeds, so make sure to rotate them in your diet. Sprinkle them on salads or eat them as a snack. Eating too many nuts and seeds at once can impair digestion, so think about just eating a small handful in one sitting.

Soaking nuts and seeds is a great way to make them healthier and tastier! Soaking helps to make the nutrients more available, improve digestibility, and reduce gut irritation. Nuts and seeds contain anti-nutrients such as phytic acid and lectins, which can impair digestion and interfere with your ability to adequately absorb and assimilate the nutrients inside. It's worth it if you have the time or if you have digestive problems!

Basic Soaking Instructions

(For a more detailed chart of soaking times for specific nuts and seeds, look online)

1. Place four cups of nuts in a glass or ceramic bowl and cover with filtered water. Add one tablespoon of sea salt and soak. (Typical soaking time is around seven hours for most nuts, but check online for the specific nut/seed.)

2. After soaking, rinse and either place in a dehydrator or on a cookie sheet lined with parchment paper to be placed in the oven. Dry at 150° F, or the lowest temperature your oven goes, for twelve to twenty-four hours, depending on the nut or seed. It's a good idea

to begin the soaking process in the morning and then put your nuts in the oven or dehydrator before bed.

Note on peanuts: Although peanuts are actually a legume, many think of them as a nut. I would recommend avoiding peanuts for a few reasons. Peanuts are one of the most common allergens, are typically heavily sprayed with pesticides, and can often contain a harmful mold called aflatoxin.

4) Quality Fats and Oils

Healthy and high-quality dietary fat is vital for a healthy brain, kidneys, and lungs; reproduction; sex and stress hormone production; cell membrane integrity; bone health; inflammation reduction; and more! Here are some examples of healthy fats/oils to eat in your diet: avocados, olives, nuts, seeds, coconut butter, coconut flakes, coconut milk, coconut oil, flax oil, hemp oil, avocado oil, grass-fed butter, and ghee.

<u>Cooking with Fats/Oils</u>

When it comes to cooking with fats and oils you've got to know your stuff. It's important to educate yourself to make sure you are eating fats and oils that are healing and not damaging to your body. There are certain fats/oils, such as the industrial seed vegetable oils, that you want to ditch all together (we will address those in the next section). And when it comes to choosing healthy fats/oils to cook with, you have to understand how to use them properly because there are varying levels of heat sensitivity based on the chemical makeup of the oil.

Fats and oils are classified into being primarily saturated, monounsaturated, and polyunsaturated. This classification system describes the chemical structure of a given fat and ultimately how stable it is. The less stable it is, the more prone it is to rancidity and the production of free radicals, which occurs by being exposed to light, heat, and oxygen.

The most stable cooking oils are saturated fats, which are typically animal fats or tropical oils like coconut and palm oils and can generally be used for cooking at medium to high heats. They are less likely to oxidize and go rancid when heat is applied. The next category of oils are monounsaturated fats like olive oil. These are typically less stable but can still be used to cook with at low to medium heat. The most unstable fats are polyunsaturated fats such as flaxseed oil. These are never to be used for cooking, are best consumed raw, typically need to be refrigerated and make good oils for salad dressings or veggie toppers.

The other consideration when it comes to cooking with fats and oils is the smoke point of the oil. The smoke point is the point at which the fat or oil begins to smoke, become damaged, and produce harmful compounds. Therefore it's helpful to know the smoke point of your cooking oils/fats so that you can use the best oil or fat for a certain desired temperature or cooking method.

For ease and simplicity, I recommend stocking your pantry/kitchen with the following five healthy fats for cooking so that you have options for high, medium, and low heat cooking.

<u>Top Five Cooking Fats and Oils</u>
1. avocado oil (monounsaturated – but has high smoke point so can be used at high temperatures) (375º–400º F)
2. grass-fed ghee (saturated – high temperatures) (450º–485º F)
3. grass-fed butter (saturated – medium temperatures) (350º F)
4. coconut oil (saturated – medium temperatures) (350º F)
5. olive oil (monounsaturated – low to medium temperatures) (325º–375º F)

Note: The smoke points listed are generalizations. The actual smoke point of an oil may depend on the individual oil/brand and whether or not it's refined or unrefined. However, it's best to always choose unrefined to avoid chemicals used in the processing of refined oils.

<u>When Selecting Quality Fats and Oils:</u>

- *Read labels.*
- *Look for these terms:* organic, unrefined, cold-pressed, expeller-pressed, extra-virgin
- *Avoid these terms:* hydrogenated, partially hydrogenated, refined, cold-processed
- *Also avoid these terms when it comes to packaged food because they often contain toxic oils:* low-fat, fat-free, reduced-fat

5) Meats and Eggs

If you choose to include some meat, poultry, and eggs in your diet, it's very important to seek out quality sources. Look for organic, grass-fed/grass-finished meats and organic, pasture-raised poultry and eggs. The food coming from these sources is *much* healthier than their conventional counterparts for several reasons. Grass-fed meat and pasture-raised poultry and eggs have a much better omega 3 to omega 6 ratio with higher levels of anti-inflammatory omega 3 fatty acids. These animals are allowed to graze, roam free, and eat their natural diet, which results in much healthier animals.

Conventional grain-fed meat on the other hand, has a poor omega 3 to omega 6 ratio (associated with inflammation) due to the high consumption of grain and soy feed they are given. Conventionally raised animals often live in poor, confined spaces (prevented from roaming and grazing) and are injected with hormones and antibiotics to fatten them up and keep them well. These are not things you want to be putting in your body! By choosing quality meats and eggs you will avoid consuming antibiotics, hormones, and pesticides and you will be getting meat and eggs from healthier animals that get plenty of exercise and fed their natural diet.

A great place to find quality grass-fed meat and pasture-raised poultry and eggs is at the farmer's market. Ask your farmer if their meat is grass-fed and grass-finished to get the highest quality meat you can find.

Some meat is marketed as "grass-fed," however the farmers finish the animals on grains at the end of their life to fatten them up, so it's good to ask. Grass-fed meats can also be accessed online these days and shipped to your door.

6) Wild-Caught or Eco-Sustainably Farmed Seafood

Be discerning when it comes to seafood. Sadly, not only are we contaminating our plants and animals on land with chemicals, hormones, and antibiotics, but we are polluting our oceans as well. Fossil fuel emissions contaminate fish with mercury, which is toxic and poses serious health concerns. However, studies reveal that selenium is protective against the negative effects of mercury and fortunately most of the fish we commonly consume contain selenium.[46]

The Monterey Bay Seafood Watch has created a helpful "Super Green List" featuring the best selections for fish based on low mercury contamination (below 216 parts per billion [ppb]), highest levels of omega 3 fatty acids (at least 250 milligrams per day (mg/d), and most sustainable fisheries. These include Atlantic mackerel (purse seine from Canada and the US), freshwater Coho salmon (farmed in tank systems, from the US), Pacific sardines (wild-caught), salmon (wild-caught, from Alaska), canned salmon (wild-caught, from Alaska).[47]

Seek out wild-caught fish and some eco-sustainably farmed seafood as long as they are fed their natural diet and raised in a way that doesn't harm the fish or environment. Most farmed fish are fed antibiotics, hormones, and genetically modified corn, and may contain dyes to make it look more appealing. Avoid these farmed fish.

Wild-caught Alaskan salmon makes an excellent choice for those on a healing path who want to include fish in their diets. It's high in the anti-inflammatory omega 3 fatty acids and contains many vitamins and minerals such as B12, vitamin D, selenium, and phosphorous.

Foods to Avoid

As mentioned, food can be medicine or can quite literally be poison and therefore it's so important to be discerning. Much of the fast, convenient, and highly processed food that the majority of people eat in our culture is devoid of nutrients and contains toxic ingredients, which is one of the reasons why chronic disease is so rampant. You will want to avoid these unnatural foods so that your body can heal. Remember, think whole, *real*, nutrient-dense food! Let's dive into the foods that you will most definitely want to avoid.

1) *Sugar*

Sugar is the first thing that must go! Sugar is one of the most damaging and inflammatory substances to the human body and many, including Dr. Robert Lustig, author of *Fat Chance: Beating the Odds Against Sugar, Processed Food, Obesity, and Disease,* considers sugar the *leading* cause of the obesity, diabetes, and metabolic syndrome epidemics. Excessive sugar consumption has been linked to heart disease, as well as markers for high blood pressure, increased triglycerides, fatty liver problems, and insulin resistance which are all indicators of potential serious health problems.[48]

From sugary soft drinks to most all refined and processed foods, we are consuming sugar in ridiculous amounts and our health is suffering because of it. Two centuries ago, the average American ate only *two pounds* of sugar a year. Nowadays, the average American consumes *150 pounds* of sugar a year – equivalent to six cups of sugar in a single week![49] That's a lot of sugar! You will find sugar in foods/beverages such as: sodas, sweet teas, Gatorade and other sugary drinks, candy, pastries, cereals, packaged and processed foods, ice cream, and many snack foods. Sugar is often snuck into many processed foods under the guise of many different names. It can get confusing so I've provided you a list here. It's important to read labels before you purchase anything and see if it contains any added sugar.

Alternative names for sugar:

- agave syrup
- brown rice syrup
- brown sugar
- cane sugar
- coconut sugar
- corn syrup
- dextrose
- evaporated cane juice
- fructose
- fruit juice concentrate
- glucose
- high-fructose corn syrup
- lactose
- malt syrup
- maltose
- maple syrup
- sucrose
- white refined sugar

2) Processed and Refined Food

Ditching the highly processed, packaged, and refined food is a must in order to get well. These are typically foods found in a box, package, or can. Sadly, these ultra-processed foods like cereal, instant soups, microwaved dinners, and packaged snack foods, make up nearly sixty percent of caloric intake for Americans.[50]

The processed food industry has become one big science experiment and by blindly consuming these foods we are the oblivious, unsuspecting lab rats. During the processing of food it is stripped of most of its nutrients and artificial preservatives and additives are added to enhance flavor, color, smell, and texture and to extend shelf life.

Nowadays, food is even manipulated with chemicals to make us more addicted to it so that we buy more! We blame our lack of self-control for consuming bags of hyper-orange colored chips that ignite a party in our mouth – but it's not all our fault. These ultra-processed foods mess with our brains and body chemistry and leave us craving more![51]

There are approximately five thousand additives allowed into our food supply and several of them have been known to cause adverse reactions. Some are outright dangerous.[52]

Russell Blaylock, neurosurgeon and author of *Excitotoxins: The Taste that Kills*, states that MSG and aspartame (two common food additives) are toxic to the brain and nervous system and have been linked to weight gain and other harmful effects on the body. Avoid these at all costs!

The take-home message here is to get rid of all highly processed food in your kitchen, fridge, and freezer. This "food" is not going to be the type of food that helps your body heal, so it's important to get rid of it. Ditch the frozen microwave dinners, instant soups, cookies, crackers, chips, cereals, frozen pizzas, etc. By getting rid of all that highly processed food in your home, you will also be well on your way to removing the added sugar since most of our added sugar intake comes from consuming ultra-processed foods.

It's ideal and beneficial if you can get your entire family on board to support you in this. It's best to remove all the junk from the pantry and fridge so that you won't be tempted to eat it. If it's not there you can't eat it! Plus, as you transition to this healthier way of living and eating you can hopefully teach your children how to be and stay healthy before they end up in your shoes with health challenges down the road.

Avoid these common toxic food additives and, generally speaking, foods with ingredients you cannot pronounce:
- artificial colors
- artificial flavors

- artificial sweeteners (e.g., aspartame, Splenda, Sweet'N Low, NutraSweet, Equal, acesulfame-K, sucralose, saccharin)
- BHA/BHT
- brominated vegetable oil
- food dyes (e.g., blue #s 1 and 2, red #3, yellow #s 5 and 6)
- hydrogenated and partially hydrogenated anything
- hydrolyzed vegetable protein
- MSG
- other preservatives and additives
- propylene glycol
- sodium nitrate/nitrate
- sodium sulfite
- soy protein isolate
- sulfur dioxide
- trans fats
- vegetable oils (e.g., soybean, canola, corn, safflower)

3) Toxic Fats and Oils

We talked earlier about the importance of consuming healthy fats and avoiding the toxic ones. This is essential to healing and being well no matter who you are. Our food supply is inundated with highly processed cheap industrial seed vegetable oils. These are toxic, inflammatory, and disastrous to your health. These oils are often the cooking oils of choice used in fast food chains and many restaurants. They are almost always found in processed and packaged foods such as frozen meals, baked goods, salad dressings, and chips.

These vegetable oils, such as canola oil, soybean oil, and margarine, are fairly new to the human diet and didn't enter the picture until the 1900s when chemical processes were invented to manufacture these cheaper, more profitable cooking oils. These oils began to replace more traditional and more expensive fats, such as butter, and were marketed as "heart-healthy" while more traditional fats were demonized as culprits in the escalating heart disease epidemic. We know now that these cheap vegetable oils are actually the ones that are incredibly inflammatory and linked to heart disease.[53]

The processing of these vegetable oils is anything but natural. These oils are heated, exposed to light and oxygen, and altered substantially through the use of chemical solvents, bleaching agents, and deodorizers to make them palatable. The chemical nature of these oils makes them very fragile and when exposed to heat, light, and oxygen they change structure and create "toxic oxidative breakdown products." These compounds negatively impact the healthy functioning of cell membranes, create inflammation, and can lead to disease in the body. These industrial seed vegetable oils are also derived from genetically modified crops, such as corn and soybeans, that are highly sprayed with pesticides.

Avoid industrial seeds vegetable oils at all costs, as well as trans fats when cooking. Trans fats are created when industrial companies add hydrogen to liquid vegetable oils such as corn, soybean, and canola oils to make them more solid (partial hydrogenation), which helps extend shelf-life. Trans fats have been linked to heart disease, cancer, autoimmune conditions, weight gain, and more. Check your labels for the list of the following oils and words such as "hydrogenated" or "partially hydrogenated." When dining out, ask what oils/fats they use to cook their food in and request that they use a more natural, stable fat such as butter or olive oil when preparing your meal.

Avoid consuming and cooking with these toxic fats:
- canola oil
- soybean oil
- safflower oil
- corn oil
- peanut oil
- cottonseed oil
- margarine
- hydrogenated and partially hydrogenated fats/oils

4) Dairy

I recommend avoiding conventional dairy entirely and most all dairy products (*with the exception of grass-fed butter and ghee) for several reasons. Dairy products such as milk and cheese can be inflammatory, gut-irritating, mucus-forming, allergenic, and may contain toxins (hormones, antibiotics and GMOs) due to the type of food fed to the animals.

Conventional milk production and factory farming uses growth hormones such as Monsanto's rBGH (recombinant bovine growth hormone) to increase milk production and profits. Exposure to these growth hormones through conventional dairy consumption can negatively impact your hormone balance and has also been linked to cancer.[54]

Many people have a hard time digesting conventional dairy due to the way it's processed (pasteurization destroys the enzymes necessary to break down the milk proteins and beneficial bacteria) and because of the presence of the complex milk proteins casein, lactose, and whey. It is estimated that seventy-five percent of the world's population is lactose-intolerant – meaning they are unable to properly digest dairy products.[55] Poor digestion and intolerance or sensitivity to certain foods creates inflammation and stress on the immune system.

Consumption of dairy products (and refined sugar) can create excess mucus production, which can lead to chronic congestion in the sinuses, ears, throat, and lungs, as well as allergies and frequent colds.[56] Ingestion of dairy proteins has also been linked to indigestion, bloating, constipation, skin rashes, arthritic conditions, autoimmune conditions such as multiple sclerosis, GERD, Crohn's, and a whole host of other conditions.[57]

Chronically elevated insulin levels can lead to insulin resistance and conditions such as metabolic syndrome, type 2 diabetes, and obesity. We typically think of sugar, refined grains, and ultra-processed carbohydrates as the main culprits in causing elevated blood sugar levels and increased insulin secretion, however dairy can as well. The carbohydrate

+ protein content in dairy causes a spike in insulin production. One study even revealed that whey (a protein found in milk) was more insulinogenic than white bread![58]

If you are dealing with any kind of chronic illness or health challenge it's best not to mess with dairy. There are too many potential issues that it's not worth it. The name of the game is to remove toxicity and things that create inflammation and stress on the body. Dairy is often one of those things for many people.

(*Note on grass-fed butter and ghee*: When it comes to grass-fed butter and ghee, the majority of the dairy proteins are gone (especially in ghee), which leaves a nutrient-dense food that contains mostly healthy fat and nutrients such as conjugated linoleic acid (CLA). Ghee is actually clarified butter, which removes nearly all protein and leaves the fat. Most people are able to eat grass-fed butter or ghee without any negative side effects, however there are those that are still sensitive. If this is the case, you may do well with ghee only or no dairy at all.)

5) Gluten and Grains

I recommend removing all gluten-containing grains, as well as keeping other grains to a minimum or removing them all together. Why avoid gluten? Gluten is a problematic protein found in grains that can be inflammatory in nature and compromise and irritate the intestinal lining. Having an intact and healthy intestinal lining and digestive system is key to being well and is a huge factor in having a strong immune system. When the intestinal lining is compromised, intact proteins such as gluten and pathogens can get into the bloodstream where they don't belong, which stresses the immune system and can be a gateway for chronic disease.

Avoid these gluten-containing grains:
- barley
- oats (you can find gluten-free oats; look on the label)

- rye
- triticale
- wheat and wheat varieties such as spelt, kamut, farro, durum, bulgar, and semolina

Grains in general are nutritionally inferior to other foods and can be problematic for many dealing with health issues. If you include gluten-free grains I would keep them to a minimum and learn to properly prepare them by soaking them to minimize anti-nutrients and gut-irritating properties. Some people do well with properly prepared gluten-free grains such as quinoa, rice, and gluten-free oats on occasion.

6) Artificial Sweeteners

I remember back in my twenties when I thought switching from Pepsi to Diet Pepsi was a healthy choice. I was cutting back on my sugar intake and making a better choice … so I thought. How horribly wrong I was! Swapping out sugar for artificial sweeteners is not a good decision and can be quite harmful for your health. Artificial sweeteners such as aspartame (Equal, NutraSweet), saccharin (Sweet'N Low), sucralose (Splenda), and Acesulfame K (Sweet One) are often touted as a healthy replacement for sugar and used to sweeten sodas, beverages, candy, and different types of processed food. Unfortunately, like sugar, artificial sweeteners are linked to excessive weight gain and an increase risk of developing metabolic syndrome, type 2 diabetes, cancer, dementia, stroke, and cardiovascular disease.[59]

Not only this, but these sweeteners over stimulate your taste receptors, causing you to crave more sugar and other hyperpalatable, unnatural foods. This excessive stimulation of taste receptors makes natural and truly healthy foods seem bland and unappealing, making it difficult to make healthy food choices. Bottom line: avoid all artificial sweeteners. Check your labels on your food and steer clear of the blue, pink, and white packets on the tables at restaurants!

7) *Processed Soy*

Conventional, processed soy is often marketed and sought after as a health food, especially by vegetarians who often consume large amounts as an alternative protein source. Once again, I was duped! In graduate school I went to Starbucks most every day to study and ordered a non-fat soy vanilla latte thinking I was being so healthy. Knowing what's healthy ain't easy, I tell you!

When it comes to soy it all depends on quality and how it's prepared. Notice here that I'm recommending avoiding processed soy, not fermented soy, which I will discuss in a moment. Processed soy is found in soy milk, meat and cheese substitutes, bagels, bread, chocolate, dairy substitutes, margarines, protein bars and powders, tofu, and many other processed and packaged foods. It finds its way into darn near every highly processed food and most all fast food in the form of soybean oil (one of those toxic industrial seed vegetables oils). It can even find its way into foods labeled as "healthy," so make sure to read your labels.

What makes processed soy a poor food choice when it comes to health? First off, soy is typically a genetically modified crop and also contains anti-nutrients or compounds that impair digestion. Secondly, in order to make the soy palatable and mask the unpleasant taste, manufacturers use noxious chemicals – bleaching and deodorizing agents. Yuck! Thirdly, according to Dr. Kaayla Daniel, author of *The Whole Soy Story: The Dark Side of America's Favorite Health Food*, there are thousands of studies linking soy consumption to malnutrition, digestive distress, immune system breakdown, thyroid dysfunction, reproductive issues, infertility, cognitive decline, heart disease, and cancer. No thanks!

Be sure to ditch all processed soy, but know that high quality, fermented soy like miso, natto, tempeh, and soy sauce on the other hand, are a completely different story. It's all about the quality of the soy and how it's prepared. Fermenting organic, non-GMO soy removes the anti-nutrients and makes the nutrients it contains easier to absorb and more digestible. Fermented soy contains vitamin K2, a nutrient beneficial for heart and bone and joint health. A bowl of miso soup, for example, can be quite healing and nourishing. Miso is a salty paste that can be made from fermented soybeans and used to make soups and sauces. Because it's fermented, miso contains live probiotic cultures or the "good bacteria" that is so important for a healthy gut and good immune function. Miso is great for improving digestion, relieving fatigue, has anti-cancer and blood pressure lowering properties, and contains several beneficial nutrients and antioxidants.

Food Quality is Key

In order to maximize your nutrition and minimize toxicity you want to focus on the highest quality, whole, *real* food that you can find and afford. Remember, quality is key. In order to avoid toxicity it's best to avoid food that contains pesticides, herbicides, fungicides, hormones, antibiotics, or food that has been genetically modified. Recall, as we've discussed in the previous chapter, the importance of reducing toxin exposure and how "toxins are the primary cause of chronic disease," according to Dr. Pizzorno.

There are more than eighty thousand chemicals used in the food supply and the accumulation and synergistic effects of these chemicals (plus toxins accumulated from water, air, and the environment) on the health of our bodies is potentially catastrophic.[60] Several of these poorly-regulated chemicals have been linked to cancers, reproductive issues, and neurological, metabolic, and hormonal problems. If you are dealing with chronic disease or health challenges of any kind, it's important to become a health detective and make wise choices when it comes to food. While we may not be able to avoid all chemicals in our food and environment, we can definitely minimize them with awareness and conscious choices.

GMOs

As mentioned, "GMO" stands for "genetically modified organism." Many people are clueless to what they are despite eating them every day – often for every meal. It is estimated that approximately 75% of processed food in grocery stores contain GMOs and the majority of the food consumed in the U.S. is processed. GMOs are also found in fast food chains and restaurants through the prevalent use of industrial seed vegetables oils derived from genetically modified crops, such as soybean oil.

Genetically modified organisms (GMOs) are created in a laboratory by taking genes from one species and inserting them into another for the purposes of obtaining a desired trait. The process is called genetic modification or genetic engineering. Genetic modification of certain food crops is currently being used in order to make these crops able to tolerate deadly doses of pesticides without being destroyed or able to produce their own internal pesticide – essentially, certain types of GMO crops such as cotton and corn are in and of themselves their own pesticide factories!

Why should you avoid genetically modified food? According to Jeffrey Smith, author of *Genetic Roulette: The Documented Health Risks of Genetically Engineered Foods,* "GMOs have been linked to thousands of toxic or allergic-type reactions, thousands of sick, sterile, and dead livestock, and damage to virtually every organ and system studied in lab animals."

Although Monsanto and huge GM seed companies will claim that GMOs are safe, there have not been long term studies on human health. GMO crops have only been present in our diets since the mid-90s. Data shows a "very strong and highly significant" correlation between the sudden increase in chronic disease occurring in the mid-90s and genetically engineered crop growth. GMO crops go hand in hand with the use of more pesticides and herbicides that these crops are designed to withstand – one of the most common and dangerous being glyphosate. When we eat these GMO foods we are exposed to these herbicides and pesticides as well. Glyphosate disrupts the endocrine system, the digestive system (the balance of gut bacteria), damages DNA, and "is a driver of mutations that lead to cancer."[61]

According to the Non-GMO Project, the highest risk GMO crops include:[62]

- Alfalfa
- Canola
- Corn
- Cotton
- Papaya
- Soy
- Sugar beets
- Zucchini and yellow summer squash

According to the Non-GMO Project the highest risk GMO animal products include:

- Meat
- Eggs
- Milk
- Products of apiculture (e.g. honey)
- Products of aquaculture (e.g. fish, gelatin, hides and skins)

Be aware that GMOs are present in many other crops and the list continues to grow – these are just the most common. Oils and products derived from these plants such as soybean oil, canola oil, high fructose corn syrup, soy protein, and soy lecithin also contain GMOs. Other sneaky ingredients that may be genetically modified include maltodextrin, natural and artificial flavors, and xanthan gum.

Genetically modified crops and the increasing use of pesticides and herbicides may be one of the big culprits in the chronic disease epidemic we have on our hands. For anyone trying to heal from any health challenge it's very important to *avoid* all GMOs!

Here's what you can do to avoid GMOs:

- Eat organic

- Avoid grain-fed, conventional meat, poultry, dairy, eggs, and most farm raised fish
- Look for food labeled with the Non-GMO Project label

Food Summary

In order to choose the highest quality foods on your healing journey, use the following strategies:

- Buy organic
- Eat whole, REAL, nutrient-dense food
- Grow your own food
- Shop at farmer's markets
- Avoid GMOs
- Use the EWG's Dirty Dozen, Clean 15 List App and online list
- Choose grass-fed, grass-finished meat, pasture-raised poultry and eggs, and wild-caught seafood
- Read labels to avoid toxic ingredients
- Shop the perimeter of the grocery store
- Eliminate all sugar
- Avoid processed, packaged, canned food as much as possible
- Avoid fast food and support farm-to-table restaurants

Digestion

It's not just about what you eat that matters when it comes to health. It's also about how well you can digest, absorb, and assimilate the food you eat. You can eat all organic fruits, vegetables, and high-quality foods, but if you aren't breaking food down properly you won't reap the benefits and you may be stressing your system.

A healthy functioning digestive system is essential to getting and being well. For us to function and live, we need our digestive system to digest our food, assimilate it (get the nutrients to the right places), remove waste, and eliminate toxins and pathogens. When working properly, it keeps the good stuff in and gets the bad stuff out. How well our bodies do this influences how we feel, our ability to prevent disease, our healing capacity, and our overall health and longevity.

So, I'm just going to say it: how often are you pooping? You should be having at least one well-formed (smooth, soft, and snake-like, and not little rabbit pellets) painless bowel movement a day. If this is not the case, you are constipated. It's important for your gut health, as well as overall health that you keep your bowels moving regularly. See the ten keys to enhance and optimize digestion below to help with bowel regularity.

Hippocrates said all disease begins in the gut. He was a smart dude. The digestive system comprises approximately seventy percent of your immunity.[63] When the gut is compromised or leaky and food and foreign particles get into the blood stream where they don't belong, it can create an immune and inflammatory cascade and be the entry point for disease in the body. Many chronic disease conditions stem from poor gut health. Functional medicine practitioners can help you to identify if you have a leaky gut and support you in resolving this. Understanding and addressing this was a huge turning point for me in my health.

Here are ten keys to enhance and optimize your digestion:

1. Drinking water with lemon first thing in the morning can jump-start digestion, get your bowels moving, and help flush out toxins.
2. Eliminate the *Foods to Avoid* (Many of these cause inflammation, gut-irritation, and toxicity to the body.
3. Chew your food until it's soup (smoothies too!). Digestion begins in the mouth. Enzymes are secreted by your salivary glands to help with breaking down food. Try chewing your food thirty-six times. The more you chew your food, the less work your stomach and intestines have to do further on down the line. Poorly chewed food is a burden to your digestive system.
4. Don't drink with meals. Drinking during meals dilutes your gastric juices and can weaken digestion. If you need to drink something with your meal, a few ounces of bone broth or hot water with

lemon is a good option. It's ideal to avoid drinking fifteen minutes before eating, during meals, and thirty to sixty minutes afterward.

5. Rest while you digest. When you are running around, eating on the go, and in a frenzied state, your body doesn't digest food well. When you are in that sympathetic or "fight or flight" state, the body shunts blood away from all necessary functions, like digestion. In order to digest well, you need to be in a parasympathetic or "rest and digest" state. Practice slowing down, eating at the dinner table with your family or friends or by yourself. Remove technology and be with your food. Take a moment to feel gratitude for your food and its ability to nourish, energize, heal, and repair your body and focus on the act of chewing, tasting, and enjoying your food!

6. Incorporate fermented or cultured vegetables such as raw sauerkraut or kimchi with your meals. Use these like a condiment. Fermented and cultured vegetables deliver good bacteria to the gut and help with the digestive process. (Note: You want to look for *raw*, unpasteurized fermented veggies, which can also be made inexpensively at home.)

7. Consider consuming quality bone broth (made from the bones of pasture-raised animals) in your diet. Bone broth contains gelatin (among other healing nutrients), which help to heal, seal, and nourish the digestive tract.

8. Move daily! Do some sort of movement every day to get the bowels moving and strengthen your digestive tract.

9. Use a Squatty Potty. The Squatty Potty is a special stool that you slide under your toilet, which allows you to elevate your feet off the floor and get your knees above the hips, which creates a more anatomically optimal angle to open the colon, allowing for full elimination of feces with ease. Unfortunately, the way toilets were designed creates a very unnatural angle for elimination and closes down the colon, which makes it more

likely you will strain and can lead to hemorrhoids, bloating, and constipation.

10. Consider taking digestive enzymes with cooked meals. Talk to your health practitioner about taking digestive enzyme with your meals to assist in breaking down your food so that you can absorb and assimilate it better.

Drink

Hydrating yourself with pure, filtered water is key when it comes to healing. Even though this is super simple, it's often overlooked. According to Dr. Batmanghelidj, author of *The Body's Many Cries for Water*, Unintentional Chronic Dehydration (UCD) produces stress, chronic pains, and many painful degenerative diseases. Your body is made of approximately 60% water and you require water to perform virtually every metabolic function in the body, so it's pretty darn important.

Here are a few tips to ensure you are adequately hydrating yourself:

- A good rule of thumb is to try to drink one half your body weight in ounces of water. This will of course vary depending on things like climate and the amount of exercise you do in a particular day. It can be helpful to track your water intake for a few days and see how much you are getting and adjust from there.

- I highly recommend finding a few glass water bottles (avoid plastic) that can hold half your body weight in ounces of water and filling them up in the morning so they are ready to go. If you do this you won't have to try to remember to fill up your water bottle or try to keep track of how much you've already been drinking.

- Drink a large glass of water with lemon in the morning to start the day off by hydrating yourself after not drinking during the night. As mentioned, water with lemon in the morning is a gentle detoxifier and helps to get the bowels moving!

- Put a pinch of high quality, unrefined Celtic or Himalayan sea salt (not refined table salt) in your water. This helps the cells and the body use and absorb the water you are drinking. Quality sea salt also contains several trace minerals.

- Include water-rich foods in your diet. Fruits and vegetables are also very hydrating. The following foods contain over ninety percent water: watermelon, cantaloupe, cucumbers, lettuce, celery, tomatoes, bell peppers, and zucchini.

Water Quality

Just like with food, water quality matters. Big time. Don't drink tap water. Invest in a water filter filtration device in order to greatly minimize toxin exposure from your drinking water. Unfortunately tap water contains a plethora of yucky stuff (over 250 contaminants in American tap water) that you don't want going into your body. While many of these contaminants fall within satisfactory levels of the Safe Drinking Act or state regulations, they are present in quantities above levels that may put your health at risk. And according to the Environmental Working Group (EWG) of these 250+ contaminants, there are more than 160 unregulated contaminants, and ninety-three are linked to increased risk of cancer, seventy-eight are associated with brain and nervous system damage, sixty-three are connected to developmental harm to children or fetuses, thirty-eight may cause fertility problems, and forty-five are linked to hormonal disruption.[64]

Possible contaminants in your drinking water could include: VOCs (volatile organic compounds) such as pesticides and herbicides, pathogenic bacteria like e-coli and giardia and other viruses, chlorine, chloramine, arsenic, aluminum, heavy metals like lead and mercury, hexavalent chromium, nitrate, and pharmaceutical residue.

The EWG has a database that will inform you of what's in your water and at what levels according to your zip code. They also provide a water filter guide that can help you find the most effective system for your individual needs based on the contaminants found in your area and your budget. There are several options for a good water filtration solution and can include reverse osmosis and solid block carbon filters, but find one that works best for your individual needs.

Drinks to Help You Heal

In addition to water, here are some of my favorite drinks that I consume daily/weekly that you may consider including in your health regimen:

- *Fresh, raw homemade juices:* Investing in a juicer to make fresh, raw juices from vegetables and fruits at home can be an incredible healing tool. Juicing allows you to consume larger quantities and varieties of vegetables and fruits on a daily basis, which have tons of healing phytonutrients, and by juicing them you are able to digest, absorb, and utilize them much easier. Juicing is a great way to maximize nutrients, boost the immune system, cleanse the body, and increase your energy.

- *Wheatgrass:* Wheatgrass is a powerhouse of nutrition. This little shot of green goodness contains anti-cancer, antioxidant, immune enhancing, and anti-aging benefits and is often recommended in natural healing protocols for a variety of conditions.[65] Just two ounces of wheatgrass contains the equivalent of five pounds of raw organic veggies. Wheatgrass packs twice the amount of vitamin A as carrots and is higher in vitamin C than oranges! It contains up to seventy percent chlorophyll and boasts the full spectrum of B vitamins, vitamin E, flavonoids, antioxidants, phytonutrients, and enzymes as well as calcium, phosphorus, magnesium, sodium, and potassium in a balanced ratio.[66]

- *Matcha tea:* I love drinking a cup of matcha in the morning and knowing I'm doing something amazing for my body. Matcha is a vibrant green tea powder that is made from grinding the whole tea leaf. It's a loaded with nutrients such as vitamin C, and contains 137 times more antioxidants than regular green tea.[67] Matcha contains high amounts of EGCg (epigallocatechin gallate), which is one of the most potent, cancer-fighting antioxidants on the planet.[68] It's also known to boost energy, induce a state of relaxed alertness, and improve focus due to its l-theanine content.

Drinks to Avoid to Heal

Avoid these beverages in order to maximize your healing potential. Alcohol and highly processed and sugar-laden drinks have no nutritional value and stress the systems of your body.

- All alcohol
- Sodas
- Store-bought fruit juices
- Energy drinks

Detox

When it comes to healing the body and keeping it well, detoxification is crucial. Chronic disease often results when the body is overwhelmed with toxicity. What happens when you don't take the garbage out or change the oil in your car? The house gets stinky and attracts bugs and your car starts breaking down and malfunctioning. Same goes for your body. The house and car need regular cleaning and maintenance and so does your body. The body gets bogged down with toxins from your food, air, water, and environment – with various chemicals, pesticides, herbicides, heavy metals, antibiotics, excess hormones, mucus accumulation, and parasites. It's ideal to incorporate daily strategies for cleansing and periodic cleanses for deep healing.

Symptoms of toxicity in the body may include:

- acne
- hormone imbalance

- body odor
- skin irritations/rashes
- bad breath
- fatigue
- constipation
- insomnia
- bloating
- headaches/migraines
- frequent illness
- puffy eyes
- inability to lose weight
- sore muscles/stiff joints

The body has a pretty amazing built-in detoxification system with seven elimination channels (colon, lungs, liver, kidneys, blood, lymph, and skin), but being bombarded with toxins on a daily basis that accumulate over time puts major stress on the body's ability to properly eliminate it. When your systems get overwhelmed they begin to malfunction, which over time can create disease in the body. It's important that you remove toxins from your food, water, home, and environments as much as possible in order to reduce exposure and to incorporate strategies to cleanse the body daily.

I also highly recommend working with a skilled holistic health practitioner who is well-versed in detoxification to properly and safely detoxify the body, especially if dealing with a complex and chronic illness. Juicing, fasting, supplement, and herbal protocols can be used to assist the body with the removal of years and years of stored up toxins that create inflammation and lead to illness.

Here are some simple, natural cleansing suggestions/techniques that require minimal equipment and investment that you may consider adding to your healing regimen. Discuss these ideas with your health care practitioner.

Cleansing Foods/Beverages

- Melons and astringent fruits such as lemons and grapes are excellent detoxifiers.
- Green juices and wheatgrass
- The following foods contain antioxidants, sulphur compounds, and/or specific nutrients that help support the liver and natural cleansing of the body: beets, sea vegetables, broccoli, lemons, garlic, artichokes, avocados, blueberries, turmeric, cabbage, kale and apples, carrots, onion, and asparagus.

Epsom Salt Baths

An Epsom salt bath is a simple and inexpensive way to detoxify the body and reduce stress. Epsom salt baths help to reduce pain and inflammation and induce a state of relaxation, which makes it a great thing to do before bed. Epsom salt contains magnesium sulfate, which helps to flush toxins from the skin and support full body detoxification. You simply dissolve two cups of Epsom salt in a warm bath and soak for about fifteen to twenty minutes. This can be done two to three times per week.

Rebounding

Rebounding involves jumping up and down on a mini trampoline and is a great way to stimulate and detox the lymphatic system. It also is known to have an immune boosting effects, improve muscle tone, and stimulate digestion. It's a great thing to do for at least five minutes in the morning to get the bowels moving and get energized for the day!

Dry Skin Brushing

Dry skin brushing involves taking a natural bristle brush with a long handle and brushing the bare skin from the feet toward the heart. You can find specific instructional videos online. This is a simple, easy way to decongest the skin (one of your detox organs), stimulate the lymphatic system, and help reduce cellulite.

Put It into Action

The quality of the food you eat and the water you drink are key elements for anyone healing from a chronic disease condition or dealing with any health challenge. Make it a priority to focus on whole, real, high-quality foods and pure, clean water. And it's not just about what you eat, but how well you can digest, absorb, assimilate, and eliminate it. Incorporate the strategies in this chapter to promote healthy digestion, as well as detoxification. Many of the things talked about in this chapter, such as eating nourishing foods, juicing, rebounding, etc. are part of my Self-Care Action Plan. Keep these things in mind when you create your own in Chapter 10.

It's time to put these suggestions, tips, and strategies into action! Go over the information in this chapter and take simple steps to upgrade your diet, digestion, hydration, and detoxification!

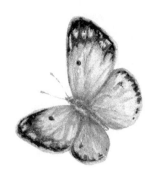

Chapter 9:

Essential #7 –
Connection and Relationships

"Only through our connectedness to others can we really know and enhance the self. And only through working on the self can we begin to enhance our connectedness to others."
– Harriet Lerner

The experience of true, authentic connection in a woman's life through life-affirming relationships (especially through sisterhood) is one of the most underestimated healing forces on the planet. On the other hand, when a woman feels isolated, disconnected from herself and others, and/or is in a toxic and depleting relationship, it negatively affects all aspects of her life and can cause her health to suffer.

There have been many gifts that have come into my life as a result of cancer. Experiencing and learning to cultivate true, authentic connection and community has been one of the greatest that I have received. It has blown my heart wide open, ushered in deep healing, and brought a richness and fullness to my life that I had not known was possible. Cultivating connection and community in my life and helping others to cultivate this has since become a passion of mine. I love to facilitate and lead women's sacred circles and provide women a safe space to connect and heal. I continue to be amazed at the power of sisterhood and how much women come alive and receive so much healing, fulfillment, and power through communing and connecting with one another.

What Is Authentic Connection, You Might Ask?

Extraordinary author and researcher Brené Brown defines connection as "the energy that exists between people when they feel seen, heard, and valued; when they can give and receive without judgment; and when they derive sustenance and strength from the relationship."

So, the question remains to be asked. Do you experience connection in your life and your relationships based on this definition? Sadly, I think there are legions of chronically sick women who are starved for connection and don't even realize it. Oftentimes, like it was for me, you don't realize it's something you've needed all along and something your heart was craving until you've actually experienced it. This was the case for Emma as well.

I met Emma at a women's circle that included about twenty women ranging from age thirty to eighty. The circle was facilitated and structured in such a way as to create a safe, non-judgmental container for each woman to share openly and authentically and to connect deeply with one another. The topic of that circle was authenticity. When we arrived, we were instructed to choose a word or phrase from the table that resonated with us at that moment in time. We then proceeded to go around the room and share why we chose the word we did.

It was Emma's turn. Emma was about sixty-five years old and was wearing a scarf that covered her bald head, was on supplemental oxygen, and had beautiful, shiny blue eyes. She said her name and read her phrase aloud:

"To Be Seen," she said meekly with a slumped posture and her piercing blues eyes glistening with tears. She proceeded to say that she almost didn't come, but she was so glad she did. She made a gesture to her scarf on her head and oxygen tank, conveying the reason why it was difficult for her to be there. "I'm tired of not being seen. I just want to be seen," she said, her eyes glancing back and forth from the floor to the group.

I thought she was finished, but to my surprise she stood up suddenly.

"I just want to be seen," she said, this time more boldly, making steady eye contact with the group, tears gushing down her face, her head held high and shoulders back as she gripped her oxygen tank. Tears welled up in my eyes and I don't believe there was a dry eye in the room.

"I see you, Emma!" my heart screamed. "I see all of you beautiful women!"

The little girl in me and the little girl in every woman in that group felt her with such intensity, because we could all relate. We all wanted to be seen too. We all wanted to be heard. We all wanted to be loved. We all wanted to feel that we mattered. That's what connection is all about. When Emma stood and boldly declared the desire of her screaming, bleeding heart with nineteen other women listening, loving and supporting her, she began to heal a deep wound that day and it was beautiful. And you know what? Her sharing created healing ripples of impact in every woman's heart that witnessed her sharing.

Although I didn't always have the language or understanding of it, I craved authentic connection and community my whole life. I believe we all do. Being an Air Force brat and having to move more often than most, I always desired a consistent, close-knit community. Looking back, I think the drive to participate in sports most of my life had a lot to do with wanting to be part of a tribe. As a social species, we are intrinsically hard-wired to connect and do life in community. Our ancestors evolved living and doing all aspects of life together in order to maximize survival and well-being. As a tribe, they would share in the responsibilities of hunting, gathering food, child rearing, and building shelter, and participated together in various cultural and spiritual rituals, singing, storytelling, and dancing. Many indigenous tribes still live this way. Living this way not only provided individuals with basic necessities, protection, and an increased chance of survival, but also the intangible benefits of connection, support, and belonging.

My husband recently returned from living amongst an indigenous tribe in the Amazon jungle of Brazil. The tribe had very little contact with the outside world, hunted and gathered all their food, and lived in huts made of trees and grasses. He was in awe at how harmonious the village was and how loving and kind the people were. They all worked so well together, everyone knowing the importance of pulling their weight, including the young children. He described how the whole village took care of each other's children, including the children taking care of the infants and was impressed by how well behaved and content the children were. He participated in their rituals, song, and dance and describes a powerful, rich and magical experience of deep connection, joy, and reverence for each other, the land, and all of life. We have lost this magic in our modern society – the magic of simplicity, connection, cooperation, celebration, reverence, and being in community with one another. We need to get our magic back.

Nowadays, we are virtually "connected" more than ever through email, social media, and the internet, yet we are more lonely, isolated, and disconnected at a heart level than any other time in history. We lack the deeper, human-to-human contact and connection that we are biologically wired to experience. There's an element of superficiality, lack of presence, and disconnect when it comes to the way we relate to people in our lives. Just take notice when you walk into a coffee shop or restaurant. How often do you see people texting away on their phones while sitting across from each other? Or how often do you catch yourself checking Facebook or Instagram while spending time with your kids, family, or friends? We are all guilty of this a time or two, but it's something to become aware of because it impairs your ability to truly connect with the people in your life. Lacking authentic connection, relationships, and opportunities where we can be seen, heard, and valued leaves us lonely and has serious implications for our health as individuals and as a collective whole.

Social connection is intimately interwoven into your mental, emotional, and physical health and well-being – likely more than you realize. Research is beginning to reveal that social isolation and loneliness are just as big of a risk factor for premature death as the more established well-known health risks such as obesity.[69]

John Cacioppo, a neuroscience researcher who has studied loneliness for over two decades, equates loneliness with starvation and dehydration – it's *THAT* important. Connection is a basic human necessity and we are robbing ourselves of it by not consciously cultivating it. In our fast-paced modern world, we need to learn to slow down and make authentic relating a priority if we want to really thrive!

Epic Loneliness

I recall about ten years ago when Chad and I had just moved to Austin. We had recently gotten married, were working as physical therapists, and didn't really know anyone. In an attempt to connect and meet people, Chad and I tried a few churches and I ended up dragging him to a co-ed church group. He knew it was important to me, so he obliged. I made and dropped off the casseroles for the women having babies and we attended every week. I tried really hard to connect, but the truth was it all felt superficial and contrived.

And then a few months into our group meetings I got really sick and we stopped going. No one called. No one came by. No one brought food. I was pretty devastated by it at the time, but I have since let it go. Chad and I struggled for the next several years, holding on to each other for dear life, sometimes wanting to strangle each other, and trying to figure out how to dig ourselves out of the deep dark abyss of suffering and sickness. I was sick at home and on disability, he was working hard to make ends meet, and we were learning how to be married and how to get over this massive hurdle. We were lonely and isolated, but grateful to have each other. As I reflect on this time, I see two dear souls doing the best that they could swirling in a sea of pain and emotions they had no tools to help them process. We were completely disconnected from ourselves and had no community support. We felt like we were drowning. It took us a long time to dig out of that crisis mode and I am certain it would have been faster if we had the support system we do now. I've been at a retreat for women dealing with cancer and almost half of the women there were left by their partners because the stress of chronic illness was too much on their relationship! To thrive we need a tribe to celebrate life's victories and to support us when life gets challenging. That's how we are meant to live.

You may be in this very boat right, now – dealing with chronic illness alone or with a partner, but the stress and weight of the situation has taken its toll. I assure you there is hope. Chad and I have been married over a decade. We now have an incredible tribe of men and women that we do life powerfully and intimately with. They are our chosen family. We do meals together, camp together, and have community gatherings by the lake where we live. We have also deepened the relationships with our family of origin and we each have intimate men's and women's circles that we connect and meet with regularly.

Chad has a circle of men that he sits and processes with every two weeks. They are his dearest brothers. When we were going through the cancer part of our journey they held space for him to express his rage and cry his tears, and supported him so he could be strong support for me. And as I write this, tears are falling from my eyes and my heart is overwhelmed with gratitude. I also have a circle of women that I meet with monthly and we are part of each other's lives daily. They are my dear sisters and there are no words to describe how much they have healed and enriched my life. Connection and community like this can be consciously cultivated and is one of the most healing and extraordinary experiences! It's clear through researching indigenous cultures and supported by modern day research that we were meant to live life connected and in community!

Cultivating Connection and Community

According to Brené Brown, "We need connection to thrive emotionally, physically, spiritually and intellectually." I agree with this whole-heartedly and I believe it's an integral component to healing and the experience of wholeness. In order to heal and live the best life imaginable, we need connection, sisterhood, and support! We need a tribe to thrive! We will talk about the power of sisterhood and developing a support team in a moment.

What Can You Do to Cultivate Connection?

1 – Take an Inventory

Take a few minutes to reflect and take an inventory of your life. How connected do you feel to others? What is the quality of your relationships? There is a saying that you are the product of the top five people you spend the most time with. Who are the five people you spend the most time with? Do they uplift you and are they supporting you in your health/life vision? Do you feel seen, heard, and valued in your relationships?

2 – Have an Intention and Stay Open

I remember several years ago when I was writing down my intentions for what I wanted to experience in my life, I wrote down this: *I have a group of women in my life who I love, trust, connect intimately with and have fun with.* I now have those women in my life and can attest to the power of intention!

What does authentic connection and community look like in your life? What would you like for it to look and feel like? If you don't have it or want to improve it, create an intention and include this in your morning ritual. Say it aloud, visualize it, and feel what it would feel like to experience it. Think and feel what it feels like when you are seen, heard, and valued and when you are enjoying time with people you really care about.

Once you create an intention, stay open and expectant. There are typically many opportunities that arise in a day or week to connect with others, but we are so closed off from the idea that we don't notice. Have the intention to connect deeper or to create new connection in your life, stay open, and watch how the Universe unfolds in your favor.

3 – Willingness to Be Vulnerable and Go First

Authentic connection requires vulnerability, plain and simple. Once I learned this, I really, really didn't like the idea of being vulnerable and I even questioned if it was really necessary. I've tested the waters and I assure you that your willingness to be vulnerable is the pathway to the connection that you desire, as well as more peace, joy, intimacy, and many of the things that you desire in your life.

If you want to connect with other people, you have to be willing to open yourself up a bit to be seen and heard and be willing to share from an authentic place. I know. It sounds scary. I was scared too. But trust me, it gets easier and the reward far outweighs the risk! It's not that you go around sharing all your innermost secrets and feelings with everyone you meet, but use your intuition and begin in small ways with someone you deem trustworthy and loving.

Have you ever had the experience of judging someone in your social circle as being perfect or always having it together? You may feel she would never like you and you've never even thought to reach out. But, what happens when you are standing in line at the grocery store together and you politely ask her how she is? To your surprise, tears start to roll down her face and she tells you she's moving through a divorce. You are stunned by her vulnerability. What happens next? Her willingness to be vulnerable begins to break down the barrier and preconceived judgments you had about her and without thinking you start to share about your divorce too. Her vulnerability makes her more human ... more relatable. The next thing you know you are hugging and planning to get tea later that week.

Understand that cultivating deeper authentic connections with people requires you to be vulnerable. I know it's uncomfortable at times, but it's a good practice to lean into that feeling of discomfort and do it anyway. Go first and start with smaller things if it scares you. You will find that it's like building a muscle. It takes practice.

Like I mentioned, I was a little apprehensive about this whole vulnerability thing at first. I was scared to put myself "out there" and afraid of what people thought if they knew the real, deep down me. I was skeptical, but I was also committed to living a heart-centered life and connection was an important piece, not to mention I wanted to be a part of a tribe or community with depth and intimacy for as long as I could remember. So, this is what I did. I decided to spend several weeks doing what I called a "vulnerability project" to see if this whole vulnerability stuff was really all it was chalked up to be and I journaled about it. First, I practiced being vulnerable in small ways. What happened during this time surprised me and was quite incredible! I shared a few tears with the plumber when he told me he had cancer, once I was willing to open up first. The hug we shared was priceless. I made a new friend at the grocery store just by genuinely asking her how she was doing and striking up conversation about the produce. I continued to have deeper, more meaningful conversations and connect with people in ways I hadn't before. It made my days feel richer and my heart more full. I couldn't believe I had the power to invite such richness into my life experience by leaning into vulnerability. And you can do it too!

Here are some ideas about how you can cultivate community and connection by being willing to be vulnerable and "go first":

- Call up a friend to schedule a coffee or lunch date.
- Host a potluck or party.
- Text a person you've always wanted to get to know better. Let them know you'd really like to get to know them better and schedule a time to chat or meet in person.

- Join a women's circle/group or start your own.
- Initiate plans for a family vacation.
- Join a local group, club, or class aligned with things that interest you (i.e. book club, gardening club, theatre group, dance lessons, pottery class, etc.).
- Ask a stranger how they are doing and listen to what they have to say.
- Speak up when you appreciate someone or something in your life.
- Tell people they are awesome and what you love about them and why.
- Ask your partner or spouse to have dinner at the dinner table, put on some music, and ask him/her all about their day and their dreams. And then listen.

4 – Make It a Priority

In this incessantly busy culture, you will have every excuse not to connect authentically with people. "I don't have time," is usually the biggest excuse. We always make time for what is important to us. And I get that perhaps up until this point you may not have thought connection was that important, but hopefully after reading this chapter you are convinced that it is! Being able to experience the fruits of connection and community takes cultivation. You must sow the seeds to reap the harvest. You've gotta take the time to be with people – to talk, love, and listen to people. There are no shortcuts.

Sisterhood Gives You Wings

As I became more and more intentional about being vulnerable and connecting with people, my heart opened more and more. It wasn't until I experienced my first taste of true sisterhood that my heart exploded and a new passion was born. The intention that I created so many years ago to have supportive, loving women in my life that I could connect deeply with finally came to fruition once I was willing to be … yup … you guessed it – vulnerable.

We had just gotten settled in my in-law's condo after moving out of our home and being on the road getting treatment at a couple cancer clinics for the past four to five months. It was good to finally land somewhere solid (thank you in-laws!) – even if it wasn't our own home. I only had a few weeks before I was scheduled for the mastectomy and I was feeling nervous about it. I did my best to prepare myself by taking walks in nature, reading, meditating, and praying. I was reading Brené Brown's book *The Gifts of Imperfection*, doing her art-journaling course, and had been learning all about vulnerability.

One day about two weeks before my surgery date, I found myself sitting outside on the porch crying. Chad was out for the evening and I was alone. Tears were streaming down my face and I felt like I was going to internally combust. I was scared and overwhelmed with grief. I was grieving the loss of my breast that was scheduled in a couple weeks, I was grieving the loss of our home, I was grieving the fact that I had tried so many things to shrink the tumor and I was still faced with having to do surgery. I felt so alone and afraid. Chad was always supportive, but he could not understand what it was like to be woman about to lose her breast. *How would this affect my marriage? My sex life? Would I have to wear different clothes? Could I wear a bikini? Would I be disgusted every time I look in the mirror?* The thoughts swam in my head like piranhas that I was sure were going to eat me alive. I was panicked to my core and terrified. I needed help. What do I do? *Vulnerability*, I thought. *Ooh … this is too personal. It's too much to share.* But, before my head could talk my heart out of it, I ran to my laptop and opened it to compose an email. In the recipient box I typed all my closest and dearest female friends – about eight of them.

Here's the gist of the email I wrote:

> *"As many of you know, Chad and I are back from the treatment center in California. We moved out of the house and now live at Chad's parent's condo. The treatment I've undergone over the past several months didn't shrink the tumor so I'm doing a mastectomy.*

I'm terrified and I need help. I don't know how to navigate this. I don't know what I need, but I need help. Thank you and I love you."
Brenda

I closed the laptop and bolted out the door and sprinted down the dark street as fast as I could until I couldn't breathe. I collapsed on the ground and sobbed until I couldn't anymore. Empty and emotionally spent, I made my way back to the house. Later that evening I got a call from my friend, Amanda. She's a lovely, warm, and gentle soul, a nutrition practitioner and healer. I picked up the phone and she said she got my email. She asked me when the surgery was and asked if she could host a healing circle for me. I didn't know what that was, but I felt a rush of gratitude and tears welled up in my eyes. "What's a healing circle?" I asked. She said to trust her and to give her the names of my other friends. We scheduled one for a few days before my surgery.

I showed up to my friend Denise's house and all my friends were there. There were candles lit, rose petals, and it smelled of essential oils. I couldn't believe they had done all of this for me. Amanda led the experience, had us all sit in a circle, and spoke some beautiful words to begin our evening together. She opened the floor to have me share what it had been like for me these past several months of being on the road. I talked and everyone listened attentively. I felt an extraordinary release to be able to have these women witness my journey over the past few months and to share my feelings that I had been largely keeping inside. It was the balm to my soul I didn't know I needed.

After I was finished sharing, Amanda had each woman go around and address me directly, sharing anything they wanted to tell me. Tears flowed down my face and my heart swelled with love for these beautiful women and the power and support of their affirming words. The circle ended with me lying on the ground and I was given an opportunity to share all my fears out loud and release them from my body while Amanda wrote them down and put them in a jar to be burned. It was one of the most healing and cathartic experiences of my life. The energy and power in that room was incredible and it is an experience that none of us will ever forget. I left that circle feeling so loved, so supported, and now had a new-found strength and the courage I needed to face the upcoming surgery. I was reminded that I am always supported and provided for. Sometimes all we have to do is be willing to ask for what we need. I walked into my surgery, headphones in, singing, dancing, and feeling the support of my sisters in my heart.

The healing circle left me reeling and desiring more connection and sisterhood with other women. A passion indeed had been born. Several of the women came to me afterwards and wanted more too. After I fully recovered from my surgery, I started my own women's circle that I still facilitate and host today. It is one of the most sacred things in my life and I am so grateful to have a group of women to do life with. These women know me inside and out. I share my fears, my celebrations, my tears, my laughter, my shadows, my scars, and my dreams with these dear souls. Each one is there for me at the drop of a hat to remind me who I am and what I'm capable of when I forget. And I do the same for them too. Sisterhood helps us all be the best version of ourselves, helps us to heal, to thrive, and gives us wings to soar – as cheesy at it sounds, it's true.

I highly recommend getting plugged into a local women's circle that focuses on connecting authentically with one another and provides a loving and safe container of non-judgment and celebrates full self-expression. Or, create one yourself! I believe that sisterhood is one of the most untapped healing powers on the planet!

Support Team

Creating a support team is critical when you are dealing with chronic illness. Sisterhood is one type of support that I highly recommend you include in your support team. Other members of your support team can include family members, friends, your partner, health practitioners of all kinds, mentors, and coaches. The key to a great support team is to have people on it who are loving, supportive, trustworthy, uplifting, have your best interest at heart, *and* are willing and able to see and relate to you in your wholeness – as your healthy, vibrant self! You want people on your support team who know your vision for your health and life and are one hundred percent on board supporting you in that vision. For example, you don't want people on your team who feel sorry for you or project fearful and negative energy and outlooks. You don't need that type of energy in your space when you are healing. If you have family members that are this way, you don't have to banish them and never talk to them again, but be mindful about what and how much you share with them. If after every time you talk to your brother or father or whomever, and they stir up fear, worry, or concern about your current health situation, then you don't need to be discussing things with that person.

I also recommend finding a team of health practitioners that believe in your body's innate ability to heal and that don't put limitations on you. Various doctors, functional medicine practitioners, nutritionists, energy workers, acupuncturists, massage therapists, life coaches, mentors, counselors, and various types of holistic healers can be great options to have on your support team. I've used a whole slew of them throughout my journey and still do. I have people on my team that support my physical, mental, emotional, and spiritual body. I've got all areas covered! You can also reach out for support for relationships and finances as well.

I find having a support team is vitally important to living my best life and keeping me healthy, strong, and in a good internal state. I always have a mentor or coach on my support team who I know can hold the Truth of who I am and reminds me of my power within to heal when I am questioning it myself, feel afraid, doubtful, or overwhelmed. How do you pick a good coach? Work with someone that you resonate with, has a loving energy (versus fearful one), and believes in the vision you have for your health and life.

Create Your Team

Create your support team by first contemplating the answers to the following questions and then writing them out on a piece of paper. Remember, your support team can consist of friends, family, teachers, mentors, coaches, counselors, trainers, doctors, support groups, women's circles, church groups, and a wide range of health practitioners. These are people that are going to support you on your path to healing and thriving. These are also the people that can and will hold you in your Truth and wholeness and support your vision and dream of vibrant health from a place of love versus fear.

- Who is currently a part of your support team?
- Is there any person(s) that does not belong on your support team that currently is?
- For example, is there someone who is extremely fearful and is constantly worried about the state of your health? You don't have to ban them from your life, especially if they are family, just be aware that this person may not be the one to call when you are having a flare-up or you are scared.
- Who would you like on your support team that isn't there already? Perhaps you could benefit from a massage therapist, a nutritionist, a women's circle, or a health coach, for example. Brainstorm ideas of people or groups that could best support you in your healing journey.

Next, take some time to assemble your team. If you've identified people that you'd like to be on your team that currently aren't, reach out and inquire or set up a time to talk or meet. For those that you have selected to be on your support team, you may consider telling them about it. It can be super helpful to clearly communicate to your people what your support team is all about and ask them if they are able to support you the way that you need. When you do this you will likely find that most people feel honored to be included on your team and it helps them understand and be clear about how they can best support you.

Relationships

When it comes to relationships they can be life-affirming and bring so much joy, richness, and love into your world, but they can also be cesspools for stress and inner emotional turmoil if we allow them to be. The good news is that we have a choice in our relationships! We don't choose our family, but we can choose how we relate to them and set healthy boundaries. When you learn to live from your heart versus your head, you will know more clearly which relationships are the ones to nurture and keep around. The quick and simple answer is – it's the ones that make you feel good (most of the time)!

Constant turmoil, drama, and toxicity in relationships, or even being in a romantic relationship that isn't your heart's truest desire, can create stressful, depleting emotions that lead to disease if they go on long enough. If you are truly committed to getting well and staying well, it's important to take a good look at the quality of your closest relationships. How do you consistently feel after you've just spent time with these people? Does spending time with these people nurture your soul, uplift you, inspire you, empower you, and encourage you? Or do you consistently feel drained, depleted, anxious, stressed, more fearful, or triggered? If it's the latter, take a good look at that relationship. You many need to create some boundaries, work on improving it with or without professional help, or let it go. Be sure to take some action on this and don't overlook it. Choosing to stay in partnerships that are toxic and depleting can make you sick – mentally, emotionally, spiritually, and physically.

If your romantic partnership is the source of immense emotional turmoil, consider getting really honest with yourself and ask your heart if he/she is the highest and best choice for you. And then take the time to listen and feel into your heart and body for the answer. I've met women dealing with chronic illness who finally get honest with themselves and acknowledge what their heart has been telling them for years – it's time to get out of that relationship and walk away. When they finally have the courage to leave the relationship after years of living with chronic pain and illness, they finally begin to heal. It's like a huge weight that had been dragging them down for years is lifted and now all the other efforts they have been making to heal could actually work. Sadly, however, many women stay in relationships that they know they shouldn't stay in because they are afraid to leave and it has very real negative consequences on their overall health.

When it comes to your romantic and close relationships, choose ones that are loving, supportive, and uplifting because you deserve it. Listen to your heart on this and have firm boundaries about the type of energy you allow into your space and your life. Don't let a relationship that isn't your highest good be a blocking factor in you getting and being well. I get that it can be hard to walk away and let go. When I reflect on past relationships that I stayed in, I see the emotional stress that I allowed for far too long. And had I been more in tune with my heart back then, I likely would've parted ways much sooner and endured much less suffering.

I highly recommend getting some professional help if needed to help you sort your feelings, especially if there is any kind of abuse happening or you've been in a long-standing marriage and have children to consider. When it comes to relationships, navigating decisions and wading through emotions can be complex and challenging. It is extremely important that you give yourself permission to get help if you need it.

Getting Complete

Getting complete with the people closest to you in your life, present and past, is one of the most healing and important things you can do. I would say if you are dealing with a chronic illness, it's crucial. Getting complete really is about forgiveness and handling any unfinished business with the people in your life. It also involves making sure the people in your life know how much you love them and how much they mean to you. If you were to die tomorrow, would you feel like you had made peace with everyone in your life? If you answered no, then it's time to make the peace *now*. Doing so will help you to release emotional burdens that you may or may not have realized you are carrying, invites deep healing, and is profoundly freeing.

Please don't overlook or skip this. You may be feeling squirmy and uncomfortable about this one, but trust me, it's worth the temporary discomfort. I get that you may not want to dig up feelings from past relationships because it might be "too painful." But, trust me, it's the working through the pain, purging of that stored up emotion, and forgiving that person that will help your body, mind, and soul find harmony and deeper healing. Recall from Chapter 6, that pain and depleting emotions like resentment and guilt stay stuck in the body and create disease if you don't deal with them and get them moving!

Focus on getting complete with your family of origin, current and past partners, friendships, or any significant relationship in your life that you still have a charge or unfinished business with (this also includes those that have passed on). A charge is an energy you feel inside yourself that keeps you from moving on from what happened or was said in the past with this person. Getting complete involves forgiveness, letting go of stored emotional energy, and feeling like you can release this person and/or situation with love from your heart and mind.

Often when you have a charge with someone it is because they did something that made you feel hurt or pain in the past and you are still hanging on. By still hanging on it's causing *you* to suffer the consequences of the emotional stress in your body, mind, and soul. You can't afford this. Holding on to shame, blame, resentment, and guilt makes you sick. Period. You may say, sure – but I'm going to need Bob to apologize to me. I didn't do anything wrong! Bob may never apologize. This is your work to find a way to forgive and get complete with Bob and let it go. Remember, forgiveness is *your* key to happiness!

Who do you need to forgive?

Previously, in Chapter 6, we talked about how doing a daily forgiveness inventory is a great way to keep depleting emotions from stockpiling. This exercise however is for you to really take inventory of your past (like yesterday or thirty years ago) and use this opportunity to let go of any unforgiveness that you've been holding on to.

First things first. Make a list. Some people/situations will be easier to forgive than others. Sometimes you will have to forgive several times and that's okay. For those particular people that you may have a harder time forgiving, you may find it helpful to talk things through with a professional or friend. It can be helpful to share your thoughts and feelings aloud in order to feel them and release them. Journaling and/or writing letters or notes to people is also very helpful. These letters can be burnt or actually given to the person. Sometimes it's helpful to actually have a conversation with a person, but not always.

I made a list and worked through it a couple years ago (and it continues to be an ongoing process as needed). My ex-boyfriend was on the list. He was the one I thought I would marry prior to meeting my husband and he broke my heart into a million pieces. I didn't realize that the last day I saw him would be the last we would spend together and I often wondered how his life turned out. He would still show up in my dreams on occasion. At the time I made my list I was happily married and grateful I didn't marry him, but I still felt an incompleteness about the way things ended. I wasn't so much angry any more, but still felt sadness and hurt, as well as gratitude for the time we spent together. I did a mini forgiveness ritual, wrote him a letter, burned it, and said a prayer releasing him and myself from any ties that bound us in time and space. It felt good. I also felt called to reach out to him via social media. I sent him a message. I told him it was an important part of my healing journey for me to get complete with all the people, now and in the past, that played an important role in my life. I thanked him for the time we shared and wanted him to know that I wished him happiness and well-being for him and his family. Once

I sent the message I felt complete. It didn't matter to me if he responded or not. He did respond, filled me in on his life, apologized, and wished me well. I haven't dreamt of him since. I felt lighter.

Who do you need to apologize to?

Is there anyone in your life that you know you need to apologize to about something (big or small) and you just haven't because you think it would be too uncomfortable or you are avoiding it entirely? If you are currently harboring guilt about something in your life this may be your indication that you may need to apologize to someone. Do it. Call the person up or write them a note. If this person isn't alive, write them a letter and burn it. You will be amazed how good it feels to clear that out of your system.

During a coaching session with Carol, she had a huge aha. She recognized that she was still holding on to an enormous amount of guilt about how she raised her daughter. She could recall to me several times that she wished she would've been less critical and more loving. She wished she would've celebrated her wins in life versus always expecting more and wished she would've listened more. She admitted she often beat herself up about this and recalled the particular events of her childhood (she was now an adult with two kids) with vivid details and she could remember the exact words she had said almost thirty years ago.

I challenged Carol to get complete with her daughter – to apologize and share with her exactly what she did with me. I encouraged her to be real and authentic, to tell her how she regretted some of the ways she acted toward her when she was a child, and to give her daughter space to share the impact it had on her. I asked Carol what new possibility she wanted to create with her. She said she deeply desired to get to know her daughter better and I could see by the tears in her eyes how sincerely she meant it. I could feel the weight of guilt she had been carrying around for so many years. I invited Carol to share this new possibility with her daughter once she apologized and they both had opportunities to share. I'm happy to say that Carol had the conversation with her daughter, and when I got to talk to her about it she was beaming and looked ten years younger. She told me that they both cried and hugged and made plans to see each other and talk more frequently.

Do all the people that you love and care for in your life know how much they mean to you?

Is there is someone in your life that you rarely tell how much you love, care, and appreciate them for what they do, what they've done, or how they show up for you in your life? I have a pretty good relationship with my younger brother, but upon taking inventory of my relationships, I realized I've never really made an effort to tell him how proud I was of him. He's created an amazing life for himself. He's kind, funny and a man of integrity. He's a wonderful dad and husband and excels at his job. I called him up and told him in detail all the ways I was proud of him. He was quite taken aback by my vulnerable sharing and was surprisingly emotional. I was floored. He told me how much it meant to him for me to say those things. I was able to let go of some guilt for not being a better sister to my brother and it made me feel so good to affirm him in a way I hadn't really ever done before. Ultimately, my act of courage and willingness to be vulnerable created healing for us both and allowed me a chance at having a closer relationship with my brother.

Who do you need to get complete with from your past and present? Your mother and father and siblings (family of origin) and partner is always a good place to start.

Again, I recommend working with a counselor, therapist, or working with a healer that does this type of work, especially if there is trauma or a significant amount of grief or pain associated with this person in your life. Forgiving this person and/or this situation is your path to freedom and essential to *your* healing. Don't make the mistake of continuing to shove it under the rug. Just make the call, schedule the time to see each other, or write a note. Quit hesitating and do it! Get complete, forgive, make amends, and move on to a life of greater peace. When you are willing to let go of longstanding unforgiveness, resentment, and bitterness it frees up energy for miracles of healing in relationships and healing of all kinds to take place.

Conscious Cultivation

When women, including myself, begin to consciously cultivate connection, community, sisterhood, a support team, and life-giving relationships we begin to transcend survival mode and really thrive. These things are often overlooked, however are essential to creating a life you love and one that is deeply fulfilling. Choosing to do so will heal and enrich your life in ways you won't know until you've experienced it. When we live life in community and connect authentically with others, we begin to experience more joy. And isn't that what life's all about? Loneliness, depression, and apathy start to fade, and we are ignited with a deep sense of belonging and well-being.

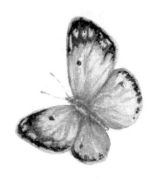

Chapter 10:

Essential #8 –
Love Yourself

"Self-love is the best medicine."
– Anita Moorjani

*"The inability to love and accept yourself and your humanity is at
the heart of many illnesses. To be loved and accepted, you must start
by loving yourself. If you have traits that you consider unlovable, you
must love them anyway ... it's a paradox."*
– Dr. Christiane Northrup

Self-love *is* the best medicine y'all. If you incorporate all the other essentials, but fail to love yourself, you will have a hard time healing and never *fully* thrive. Loving yourself and your life may be the single most important thing any woman desiring to heal her body can do. We've already talked in previous chapters about the power of your thoughts, words, feelings, and beliefs. What is the narrative inside your head when it comes to the topic of *you*? What do you believe about yourself? What do you say to others about yourself? How do you feel about yourself? These are all important questions to explore and ask yourself. It's so easy to get caught up believing and identifying with the voice in your head telling you that you aren't enough, that you're ugly, stupid, too fat, too thin, or that you'll never get better. Unfortunately, we all have some version of these voices, but it's your work to call them out for what they are – lies – and let them go. These voices aren't true and they aren't *you*! It's time to choose compassion and love for yourself instead. Why? Because you are magnificent. Because Love is who you are and why you are here. And because Love is the vibration in which you heal.

When I was in California I'd spend full days Monday through Friday at the healing center getting treatments and afterwards I would go to the beach as often as I could. It was my sanctuary. I would stroll for hours picking up sea glass and watching the waves crash on the shore. There was one moment on the beach that I'll never forget. I was walking along the beach and glanced over at the water and saw millions of diamonds sparkling on the surface of the water as the sun hit the water just right. It sounds strange, but it felt like a gift just for me. "You are magnificent," said the soft whisper in my heart. I was taken aback. I furrowed my brow and looked around.

Who, me? I thought. I started to think I was foolish and must've been mistaken.

"Yes," the whisper said. I smiled and a rush of warmth and an indescribable sense of love filled my body as I stared at the sparkling ocean. I hadn't felt anything quite like it before. It was the moment I started to remember how magnificent I was – how we all are. It wasn't a cocky thing by any means, it was just Truth that I had forgotten long ago. It's something that we all knew when we were infants, we just forgot somewhere along the way.

Babies know their magnificence and revel in it fully without reservation or self-criticism. They express their laughter, their pain, and their fury the moment it arises. They exude joy and curiosity and marvel at life. They do not question their worth or their awesomeness until they grow up and learn to think otherwise. Babies just *are* their unique, magnificent selves. We were that way once too. That is who we really are too and it's crucial that we remember that little child inside each of us. Somewhere along the way we forgot that we were extraordinary, magnificent divine manifestations of the Infinite and it's costing us our health, happiness, and our lives. The forgetting of this is a monumental error. Healing is about remembering and reclaiming this Truth.

There is a teaching from Jesus in the book of Matthew that says, "Truly I tell you, unless you change and become like little children, you will never enter the kingdom of heaven." Regardless of your feelings and beliefs about Jesus, this is a profoundly wise teaching and invitation to healing and wholeness. I have come to understand the "kingdom of heaven" as a state of pure love consciousness that can be accessed in the here and now. It's the state of love, peace, and joy that we all crave, because that is the very essence of who we are and what we were created for. Jesus reminds us that to achieve this state we must become like little children. We must remember our magnificence.

Can you think back to a happy, joyous moment when you were a young child? When you felt fully alive and free? What were you doing and how were you feeling? I have a memory of myself playing arts and crafts with my mom. I had a huge smile on my face, wide-eyed and bubbling with excitement and creativity. I was making all kinds of things out of Play-Doh and loving every moment. This little girl is who I am. And whatever little girl you conjured up in your memory … that's the real, true you! She's still there inside you waiting for you to love and nurture her.

In my memory there was no self-doubt. No, "mom, do you think this is okay?" No self-condemnation. "It's horrible, I need to start over!" And no self-criticism. "Well, this is okay, but it would've been better if I'd given the Play-Doh snowman a different hat, don't you think?" Ahhhh! But, isn't this how we talk to ourselves as adults, constantly doubting and criticizing ourselves and actually believing it all? Sadly, we've spent a lifetime being programmed by our culture and surroundings that we are not enough and that somehow we must figure out how to earn the love that is already inside us. We've been led to believe we are broken, unlovable, and undeserving. The healing process involves letting go, unlearning, and casting away these lies.

Remember from Chapter 5, how we talked about the importance of being an avid gardener of your mind? Make a commitment not to tolerate those self-critical, fearful, and condemning thoughts about yourself that multiply like weeds if you let them. Those thoughts aren't you and aren't true. Don't push them away, just use them to alert you to shift back to thoughts of loving kindness and activate those core heart emotions of love and gratitude. Historically I've struggled with being very critical of myself. I have a quote next to my bed that reminds me to be compassionate with myself and always serves as a great reminder for me to soften and be more loving. Consider putting quotes and affirmations like this by your bed, on your desk, on your mirror, and other places where you can see them.

Begin to think about these questions: How can you love and accept yourself more fully? How can you speak to yourself more lovingly (aloud and inside your mind)? How can you care for yourself in a loving and kind way? How can you find more joy in your life as it is in this moment? We think we will start to love ourselves and enjoy our lives once we get better, but ironically, it's in the loving and accepting ourselves and this life *now* that is the pathway to feeling better and moving beyond our current circumstances.

You Are a Queen

"At every moment, a woman makes a choice: between the state of the queen and the state of the slave girl. In our natural state, we are glorious beings. In the world of illusion, we are lost and imprisoned, slaves to our appetites and our will to false power. Our jailer is a three-headed monster: one head our past, one our insecurity, and one our popular culture."
– Marianne Williamson, *A Woman's Worth*

We went to visit some dear friends of ours who have two kids, one of them being an eight-year-old little girl named Brianna. We see them about once a year and I love them like they are my family. I enjoy watching the kids grow and change and hearing about what they are learning and what excites them. Brianna is pure joy and lights up a room. She is kind, bubbly, creative, confident, and full of life. She dances, she sings, she twirls, and makes up stories. Being around her wakes up the carefree little girl spirit within me and we play, dance and sing together – I cherish every second of it.

However, this trip she seemed a bit different to me … still kind, bubbly, and creative, but something was "off." Jenny, her mother, mentioned she has been going through some changes and was more emotional lately. Jenny and I were chatting at the table and noticed Brianna was crying in the den. Jenny left to go see what was wrong and returned fifteen minutes later exasperated and confused.

"She is worried she is getting fat," she said.

"What?! … that's crazy!" I exclaimed. My breath caught in my throat. *No! No, no, no, no. She's absolutely perfect and beautiful and innocent*, I thought.

"No! She's too young to even be thinking about this, right?" I said.

"I know!" her mom replied. "I don't know where she is getting this stuff from."

Later in the day I went to her room to spend time with her. Her room is full of pink and purple princess garb, puppies, and horses – all the things that little girls love. I asked her about her comment she made earlier about worrying she was getting fat. I asked her to tell me more about how she was feeling. She said, "When I look in the mirror I see that my cheeks are fat and I'm worried the rest of me will get fat."

My heart sank into my stomach and tears welled up in the corner of my eyes. How could such a young, innocent, beautiful little girl think she was anything but amazing? I felt simultaneous sadness and anger. I could relate to these self-critical and judgmental thoughts and feelings she was having. But, did I have them when I was so young? I was just shocked at how early girls begin to feed into these lies of "you're too fat" or "you're not good enough." When we hear or are around this enough we begin to believe it. These messages of criticism, insecurity, unworthiness, guilt, shame, and negativity are lurking everywhere and we absorb them like osmosis, especially when we are young. As young children we pick up on what is said and modeled by our families, by the women we look up to (whether they realize it or not), by our pop culture, and by the way in which women have been perceived and treated throughout history.

"Oh honey – You are so beautiful! Your cheeks are perfect and so is your body," I said.

"But, I understand how you feel. Sometimes I look in the mirror and don't like what I see. Sometimes we fall into the habit of comparing ourselves with other people – friends, models, movie stars – and we think we are not enough. It makes us criticize and judge ourselves. But, those silly voices in our head – they aren't telling the truth. The truth is that you are beautiful and perfect just the way you are – I promise. When those voices come in my head, I have to remind myself that the truth is usually the opposite!"

"Really?" she said.

"Yes. Those voices aren't telling you the truth. The truth is that your cheeks are adorable and perfect." And I tickled her.

"Okay," and she giggled and squirmed. She seemed appeased and asked me to help her pick out her outfit for the day. The heaviness of the moment seemed to have melted away and the glorious queen (or perhaps the princess!) emerged again (at least for now).

Despite how you were raised, all the things you've done or gone through in the past, or the culture in which we live, you have a choice in who you will be. At any given moment you can choose to be a slave girl or a glorious queen – it's up to you. It is in the letting go of the past and what other people think and learning to love ourselves that we can free ourselves from being slaves and reclaim our royalty. We must become attuned to the inner critic and not let those outer critics shake us! Is your inner critic telling you that you are stupid? Is your partner telling you that your dream is unreasonable? Do you have a tape of your mother's voice inside your head telling you that you're chubby? Remember, the mind will always have things to say, but we have a choice whether or not we choose to believe it and can replace those thoughts with true and loving ones.

The truth is that you are whole, beautiful, strong, fascinating, and brave. You are dearly and deeply loved. If you don't believe this yet, that's okay. Somewhere, perhaps buried deep down inside you, you know this is true. Sometimes the unlearning of the lifetime of lies you've been told about who you are takes time to unravel like it did for me. It can be a process. Rest assured your soul is beckoning for you to reclaim your knowing of yourself as the queen that you are and is one of the most healing and loving things you could ever do.

Self-Care

In order to begin to love yourself again and own your queen status, it's time to care of you! It's time to love *you*. So often as women we care for everyone else's needs but our own and become extremely depleted, exhausted, often resentful, and sick in the process. Not only is making self-care a priority essential to healing and loving yourself and your life, it helps you decrease stress, brings you joy and lifts your mood, improves relationships, and helps you make better decisions and become more resilient. When your cup is full and your inner battery is charged, you will be able to give and serve your family and the world from a full heart in such a way that doesn't make you depleted or sick.

Self-care involves not only caring for your body, but your mind, heart, and soul too. Take a moment and consider how well you care for yourself physically, mentally, emotionally, and spiritually. Most women engage in some degree of self-care for themselves physically. They may be trying to eat healthier and exercise. Nutrition and exercise are great foundations for a good self-care plan, but for any woman dealing with chronic health challenges (or any women wanting to thrive) you've gotta dig deeper. So many women neglect caring for themselves mentally, emotionally, and spiritually. As you create your Self-Care Action Plan be sure to incorporate things that support and nourish all aspects of yourself.

Creating a Plan

You must be intentional about caring for yourself and creating space in your schedule in order to make it happen. I highly recommend creating a Self-Care Action Plan. Your plan will include things that you do daily, weekly, or monthly to prioritize taking care of your body, mind, heart, and spirit. This is something I have all my clients do and it helps lay the foundation for healing and thriving!

What nourishes you?

Create a list of things you know that are important in taking exceptional care of yourself. Perhaps these are things that you have pushed by the wayside because there's not "enough time." Newsflash, we *always* have enough time for what's important to us. There's nothing more important than your well-being. I know some of you will be saying that your kids are more important. Your kids deserve a mom that loves and cares for herself. Your kids learn by watching and mirroring you. Think about what things are required to nourish your body, mind, heart, and spirit. Several things will overlap, of course, but here are some examples and recommendations of what you could consider including. Consider the previous essentials we've discussed, as well as things that really nourish you, and include them as part of your self-care plan. For example, bubble baths might be something that really relax your body and mind and really nourish you. Put it down! Perhaps you could schedule a bubble bath once a week or once a month!

Here are some ideas and recommendations for your Self-Care Action Plan:
Daily:
- Meditation

- Say intention aloud
- Use your Whole-Hearted Vision book for activating imagination
- Glass of water with lemon upon rising
- Fifteen to thirty minutes of movement/exercise
- Freshly made juice
- Eating healthy, nourishing food each meal
- Be in nature every day
- Daily dose of sunshine, thirty minutes
- Do one thing from my joy list (I'll explain this later in this chapter)

Weekly:
- Journaling
- Dancing a couple times a week in my living room
- Goddess date bi-weekly (I'll explain this later in this chapter)
- Use a gentle detox strategy three times per week (rebounding, detox bath, sauna, or dry-skin brushing)
- Play with dog
- Yoga two times per week
- Light resistance training two times per week

Monthly:
- Attending monthly women's circle or group
- Massage, energy work, or acupuncture one time per month
- Do something more involved from my joy list one time per month
- Ride my bike twice a month
- Meet with my coach/mentor one time per month

Once you have your list, look at your current schedule and figure out when you can make these things happen. When will you meditate? For how long? When will you exercise? It's important to block out time for your self-care so you can ensure you make it a priority. If you are not currently doing any of these things and it feels incredibly overwhelming, start with one thing, implement it successfully for a few days to a week, and then do the next one. Just remember, it's so important to create a plan that will nourish your body, mind, heart, and spirit!

Saying No

Sometimes (or oftentimes) self-care means saying a very tiny, but transformative word – *no*. I know, this may be incredibly challenging at first, but trust me, if you want to get well and love yourself again you've got to stop saying yes to every request, opportunity, and demand that comes down the pipeline. People pleasing or saying yes when our hearts and bodies tell us no is precisely what leads to stress, exhaustion, unhappiness, and sickness. It could be as simple as saying yes to the request to join the PTA, yes to hosting the cocktail party for your husband's VIP clients, yes to dog sitting the neighbor's brand-new puppy for the weekend, and yes to volunteering at the church each week (in addition to your full-time job) that has led you to your current point of sickness, exhaustion, and overwhelm. Why did you say yes to all these things? The common answer I get is "well, I have to" because that's what a nice person does, a Christian woman does, a good mom does, a good wife does, a good neighbor does … etc. These are responses based on your current beliefs and your desire to look good, avoid looking bad, and please other people. You don't "have" to do any of those things, but you did choose them and you can choose to say no as well. When you begin living and leading with your heart you will learn to ask your highest Self what to do and respond yes or no accordingly. This is living from your authentic self instead of living your life based on what other people think you "should" do. When you make decisions aligned with your highest Self, life gets much easier and more fulfilling and you begin moving toward that place of wholeness.

Start practicing saying "no" and experience the freedom that comes with it. Your health may very well depend on it. People in your life may be so used to you saying yes to their every call and request, that they may be taken aback or respond negatively to your refusal. Don't let that deter you. Give them time to readjust to the new empowered you. The people in your life that truly love you will continue to love you, respect you, and often trust you more for being aligned with your truth.

When asked to do something, take on a new project, or go to an event and you aren't sure if you really want to, say something like:

"Thank you for the invite or opportunity. I am not sure if I'm able to do that, can I get back to you tomorrow or by this weekend?"

Or

"Thank you for the invite or opportunity. I have several projects on my plate right now and I need a little time to feel into whether or not I'm able to do this, can I get back to you tomorrow or by this weekend?"

Give yourself some time to check-in with yourself to see if it's something that is a true "yes" for you or not. Also, don't be afraid to just say, "No, I'm not able to do that at this time. But, thank you so much for thinking of me!" You don't have to give a reason. Most of the time people will give you time to make a decision and you can use that time to check in with yourself and get back to them with a decision that's right for you. If they need a decision right away and you aren't sure, I recommend saying no. Just decide that "no" is your default when those situations arise and then you already know what to do! This way you don't get schmoozed into something that's going to cause you to expend way too much energy that you don't have and end up regretting it.

When you stay true to yourself by saying no when you mean no, your yeses will be empowered yeses and the choices you make will enrich your life and be in alignment with helping you heal and a create a life that you love.

Follow Your Bliss

What lights you up?
What makes your soul come alive?
What makes you feel joy?
What gives you pleasure?

What do you do (or what have you done in the past) that makes time stand still or fly by?

Take the time to contemplate these questions. Find out the answers for yourself and *do* them. Trust me, a happy and joyful heart is powerful medicine. Do not be disheartened if you do not know! The fun part is discovering or rediscovering this for yourself. That's where a Joy List comes in handy.

I mentioned in Chapter 2 a time in my healing journey when one of my mentors asked what I loved to do and I could not respond because I honestly didn't know. I had spent the majority of my life living for other people and attempting to be successful in the eyes of the world. Living this way left me unfulfilled and I know it negatively impacted my health. I had failed to stop and really ask myself what *I* loved to do. You may be able to relate. In order to begin to cultivate more joy in my life I began brainstorming and creating a simple list of all the things that brought me joy and started actually doing these things daily. I was so amazed at how my life began to feel so much more joyful and rich. It's one of my favorite exercises and one of the most fun things I do with my clients. I love watching women find their joy again. It's a beautiful thing and is an integral part of your self-care, self-love, and healing regimen.

I had a client named Mary. She was dealing with a neurological condition that modern medicine deems "incurable." When we first met she had a significant amount of fear and sadness about what the future would hold for her. Would she lose her ability to walk without assistance? Be unable to hike in nature? End up in a nursing home unable to care for herself? All of which are totally understandable fears. However, the fear was keeping her from healing and keeping her from fully living. I had Mary create a Joy List. I found out that Mary loved to dance and was a dancer when she was younger. She loved to swim. She loved to paint. She loved to kayak. I asked her if she was doing any of these things and she said, "no." When I asked her why she said she wasn't entirely sure and that perhaps when it came to kayaking, she was afraid of losing her balance in the kayak. It's fascinating and unfortunate how fear can suck the joy out of our lives. I gave her homework. Each day she was to do something that brought her joy.

By the end of our time together she was a different person. She exuded a completely different energy. She was much more joyful, calm, and confident. She started painting again, she planned a family dance party for her fiftieth wedding anniversary, she kayaked with her husband, she made plans to hike the Grand Canyon. She was no longer suffocating under the weight of a diagnosis and letting that keep her from enjoying her life. She began fully living and loving her life. It was beautiful to witness. It's quite incredible what following your bliss can do!

Creating Your Joy List

Here's how you do it. Get a piece of paper out and draw a line down the middle. On one side put the heading "Things that cost money" and on the other side put "Things that don't cost money." Now, begin brainstorming and write your ideas in the appropriate columns. If you have some ideas, but you don't know if you will like something or maybe it's something that you always wanted to try but haven't, put those things on there. For example, for many years I thought I might enjoy organic gardening. I liked the idea of growing my own nutritious food, so I built an organic square foot garden. I bought a book online, went to Home Depot and got the wood, drill, and supplies. I'd never used a drill in my life and I actually built a wooden garden all by myself! I planted the seeds and the starters. I put a lot of sweat equity into that little guy and was so proud to get my first summer squash. It brought me so much joy to accomplish such a thing on my own. But, then because I didn't know too much about organic gardening, the pesky Texas bugs decimated my entire garden before I could get much yield out of it. I decided that it was a great experience, but I didn't love gardening. I decided to stick with going to the farmer's market to get my food, at least for the time being. Maybe I'll try again when I learn a little more, but it was a fun adventure and I learned how to use a drill!

Hold nothing back as you create your joy list. Include small and big things and things that you aren't sure of but would like to try. Use the list you create and pick one thing to do every day that brings you joy. It can be as simple as drinking tea from your favorite mug while sitting on the balcony and watching the birds or buying yourself flowers, or more involved like going to a symphony. Plan ahead for the more elaborate activities and trips. Do you love the beach, but you live three hours away? Plan a beach trip in the next six months. Just the act of starting to plan your getaway will bring you joy.

Goddess Date

One way to be exceptionally intentional about cultivating joy and loving yourself is planning a weekly or bi-weekly goddess date or royal respite. This is your time to fill your love tank, pamper and enjoy yourself, and spend time alone with the amazing *you*. Goddess dates do wonders for filling a woman's cup, nourishing her soul, and helping her re-connect to herself, and are profoundly healing.

An example of a goddess date might be something like this. On Thursdays, when you come home from work, you lock yourself in the bathroom and draw a bubble bath. Get some soft music playing. Set a timer and soak in the tub for thirty minutes. Take the time to lovingly wash your body with appreciation – thanking your body parts for all their hard work today and over the years. Sing if you please and enjoy yourself. Finish your time by applying massage oil to your body, spending extra time on areas that are sore and need a little more love. Dress yourself in some beautiful, comfortable clothes that make you feel good and return to the household to reconnect with your partner or family. How much different do you think you will feel and act after taking that time to nurture yourself? After feeling more relaxed and grounded, you are much more likely to be the partner and mother you desire to be.

Shifting your energy to a more calm and joyful place allows you to be the best version of yourself and almost always infuses your entire home and the people around you with that same energy. I'm telling you, goddess dates can work magic!

Here are a few other goddess date ideas, but the possibilities are endless!

- Take yourself on a date to an art museum you've always wanted to see
- Treat yourself to shopping for a new dress or sexy lingerie
- Try a pottery class
- Take a dance class that interests you
- Go see a movie
- Get a massage or some type of body work
- Take thirty minutes to do yoga and have time away from the kids

Fall Back in Love with You

I believe that *not* loving ourselves and knowing our worth as glorious and magnificent queens is one of the main underlying culprits of chronic illness. Falling back in love with yourself invites healing and the experience of wholeness to take place. As you move forward from this moment on, remember (and remind yourself as much as it takes) that you are a magnificent queen and begin to love and care for yourself accordingly.

Be sure to plan out your self-care routine and make it a priority to nourish your body, mind, heart, and spirit. Realize that you have the power to choose what you do with your time. Don't forget that saying no may be one of the biggest tools in your healing toolkit. Use it and begin to make decisions from your heart, not from your head. Follow your bliss and take time to cultivate joy every day. Joy is what makes life worth living. You have the ability to infuse your life with the healing power of love and joy, so choose it! Choose to live and love fully *now*.

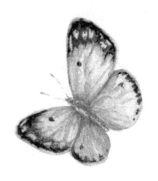

Chapter 11:

Essential #9 –
Trust and Surrender

"Always say 'yes' to the present moment. What could be more futile, more insane, than to create inner resistance to what already is? What could be more insane than to oppose life itself, which is now and always now? Surrender to what is. Say 'yes' to life – and see how life suddenly starts working for you rather than against you."
– Eckhart Tolle

The path of true healing, wholeness, and freedom from suffering is one of surrender. Surrender invites us to accept the moment or circumstance as it is, to let go of holding on so tight, to be okay in the not-knowing, and to trust that Divine Intelligence will provide all the answers we need and always has our highest and best interest at heart. When you are experiencing difficult health challenges, it's so easy to get sucked into the vortex of trying to control the situation, to understand it, to resist it or figure it all out on your own. So much energy is wasted here, causing us to suffer and keeping us stuck in a place of fear. Instead, we can choose to surrender. We can surrender the pain, surrender the diagnosis, surrender that fear, surrender the decision, and surrender day by day, moment by moment. To surrender requires trust and faith that God's got your back. I know it sounds scary and maybe super uncomfortable at first, but it is surrendering that frees us and allows us to open to receive the guidance, healing, and peace that we are seeking.

Remember when I got the message that I needed to learn listen to my heart after I found the lump in my breast? I was grateful for the message, but scared and worried because I didn't know how to listen my heart. I wondered if I could trust my heart to guide me when the stakes were so high. In my quest to uncover just how to listen to my heart, I learned that listening and trusting the heart also went hand in hand with surrender. All the healing and spiritual books and gurus said so. I kept hearing "to heal you need to learn to let go and surrender." *Okay, great,* I thought, *but, what the heck does that even mean and how do I do that?!* The books and gurus spoke of the importance of having faith in God and trusting and surrendering to my Higher Power within to guide and heal me. It sounded so simple, yet in my brain it seemed so complex and inaccessible. I was so used to trying to figure out everything myself, I wasn't sure how to completely surrender.

I've always believed in God, but I don't think I ever *really,* truly trusted God to lead and guide my life. I'd been trying "my way" for eight years and here I was in a precarious pickle of a situation. It was time to try something new. I agreed to give this whole surrender thing a try. Plus, I was tired of trying so hard – bone tired – of trying to figure it all out on my own. I wanted to learn to surrender and trust my heart, to trust my body to heal … to trust that God would provide all I needed in every given moment. I wanted to, I knew I needed to, but I didn't exactly know how.

I kept trying to wrap my mind around this whole "surrender" thing because I couldn't quite make it gel. So, I did what I always do, and found a book on the topic in hopes it would help me. Okay, so in a moment of transparency, I read the whole book, closed it, and *still* didn't "get it." I kept anticipating and waiting for the step-by-step, 1-2-3 process on how to surrender, which never came. After completing the book I turned to my husband and said, "There is no step-by-step guide on how to surrender in this whole book." He smiled affectionately and laughed and said, "Oh honey, you just let go. It's not a head thing, it's a heart thing. It requires trust." Ugh (sigh). There's that heart thing again.

Over the next year or so, I focused on getting more in touch with my heart by cultivating qualities of the heart like love, joy, compassion, courage, and connection. I slowed down and made time to listen to my heart and love myself more fully. I learned to harness my power to heal by beginning to let go of limiting beliefs, thoughts, words, and feelings and began to think and feel greater than my circumstances. I started to shift my thoughts, beliefs, words, feelings, and actions in alignment with my dreams of health and happiness and did so from a place of surrender and trusting that God always has my best interest in mind. I gradually began to learn what it meant to surrender and to flow with life. It is glorious when I am able to fully surrender in this way. I feel much more freedom, peace, and love. This continues to be an ongoing practice for me. I'm definitely not perfect at this by any means. I still catch myself getting caught up in trying to control my life, to fix or force things, and get swept up into fear. The dead giveaway that I'm not in a state of surrender or flow is when I feel angst, disconnected, worry, overwhelmed, or confused. I use these feeling states to remind me to surrender once again. I find that it's also helpful for me to talk to a coach or mentor when I get stuck in a place of fear, forcing, fixing, and trying to figure things out on my own, which also helps me to find my way back to my heart. Living this way really is a choice. The more we cultivate practices of self-awareness and connect with our hearts, the better we are able to make powerful and loving choices for our lives.

The Alchemy of Surrender

Here's a powerful example in my life of what's possible when choosing to surrender in the moment:

Making the choice to have a mastectomy was one of the most challenging decisions of my life. It was challenging because my heart was telling me to do it, but my head was screaming "no!" The voices in my head told me that having the surgery meant I failed and spoke of all the things that could go wrong. I went forward with it because I made a solid commitment to following my heart and I was learning to trust and surrender.

When I told my parents about my choice to have the surgery, it was just a "given" that my mom would travel here to be with me for however long I needed – because that's just how awesome my mom is. Having her here with me before, during and after my surgery, meant so much to me that I can't even put it into words. She spent the night with me in the hospital and was there to comfort me when I woke up in the middle of the night with searing pain in my chest. I've never felt more relieved in my life to see her there. Together we ate homemade Jell-O (made from organic fruit and grass-fed gelatin of course!) that my mom made and brought to the hospital and watched a movie at 2 a.m. until we both fell asleep. The next day she drove me home.

Once we were home she cared for me like only mothers can. She made me soups from scratch, special healing drinks, emptied my surgical drain, propped me up with pillows until I was comfortable, kept me company, made me laugh, and thought of all the little details without me having to ask.

After a few days, it was time for me to take a shower. Since even before the surgery I was dreading the part where I would have to see my massive scar and barren chest for the first time. When the time came I had knots in my stomach. I needed some help with the shower because I still had a plastic drain that exited my ribcage to drain the fluid and it was difficult to hold it while washing myself. My mom came with me downstairs to help, but I asked that I go in the bathroom alone to unwrap the bandage. I was nervous and I didn't know how I was going to feel, seeing that my breast was no longer there. I went in the bathroom and closed the door. My mom stayed right outside in case I needed her.

I turned Pandora on from my phone to a relaxing music channel and the melodies flooded the silence. I welcomed the soothing sounds to calm my nerves. I stood in front of the mirror and slowly unwrapped the bandage from around my chest. I looked at my reflection and my eyes immediately welled up with tears, my throat and chest tightened, and I had trouble catching my breath. *How horrible … how barbaric … what did I do?!* The voices in my head screamed. A couple tears streamed down my face. As I was about to give way to the agony and self-pity … I heard in my heart a stern but a loving *No, you've cried enough tears, my love.* And then the song "Let It Be" by the Beatles came on in perfect, divine timing and spoke directly to my soul.

I smiled and I could feel the shift … the sweet surrender. I heard, *"You are beautiful and perfect exactly as you are … Let It Be."* I felt all the anguish, disgust, and pain melt away in an instant.

I turned from the mirror and stuck my head out the door. I asked my mom to help me shower. She came in to help me. As she looked at me in my breastless state with my four-inch scar, I searched her eyes for disgust but I could find and feel only love. After the shower, I sat on the vanity seat while my mom re-bandaged me. She brushed my hair and began to braid it and my mind drifted to when I was a little girl. I felt a surge of love and tears welled up in my eyes again. I felt an immense amount of gratitude for her being there and getting to share this moment with her. I marveled at the incredible shift from intense anguish, judgment, grief, and self-pity to surrender, gratitude, acceptance, and love in such a short time.

I can't remember a time I've ever been so grateful or felt such an overwhelming love for my mother than this experience with her. I'll never forget this memory. It will always serve as a vivid reminder of the alchemical power of surrender to turn something I thought was so horrible into "gold." There is always gold or a gift available in the midst of our most difficult times and perceived challenges. Surrender is the portal to returning to peace in the moment and experiencing the gold and the gifts waiting for us to receive them.

I could've stayed in the place of self-loathing and fear. No one would've blamed me for it. It was completely justifiable. However, which state is the one more conducive to healing? Which state allows me to experience more of what I truly want – love, peace, joy, and connection? Is it the place of self-loathing and fear and thoughts of *"You idiot – what did you do?"* and *"Why did this have to happen to me?"* Or is it accepting what is and experiencing the gift of fully receiving in my heart the fierce and gentle love of my mom and the overwhelming amount of gratitude – a memory that I will cherish for the rest of my life? Love always wins. Love heals every time. The more fully we love ourselves, love our lives, love what is, and surrender fully to the moment, the more healing and wholeness we experience. It's important to remind ourselves to not be so quick to label things as "good" or "bad." There are seeds of grace, nuggets of gold, and incomprehensible gifts in every situation if we stay open to receive them.

Intuition and Making Decisions

Here's what I know for sure. Every day you will have decisions to make about your health and life. And, every single person's healing path is different. There aren't two alike. What "worked" or is helpful for one person may not "work" or be helpful for another. When you are dealing with a chronic health problem and you desperately seeking the answers to your dilemma outside yourself or expect someone or something to fix you, that which you are seeking will elude and exhaust you. The answers truly are within you and are accessed through your heart. Your intuition is the extraordinary GPS or guidance system within you – that "still small voice" of God and subtle knowing that is constantly directing and guiding you toward your highest good if you choose to listen. It's always been there, but we've learned not to trust it and some of us have completely drowned it out by the chaos in our minds and lives. In order to begin to learn to hear that voice within, we must learn to slow down and trust our Self.

Have you ever been in a situation where you needed to make a decision and you had a "gut feeling" to do one thing, but it didn't really make logical sense so you ignored it and followed your intellect instead?

Perhaps days, weeks, or months later it became very clear that you didn't make the best choice and wished you would've listened to that "gut feeling"? You've likely had several instances of this occurrence in your lifetime. This is your intuition and it's time to get reacquainted! Why? It will help guide you on your healing journey and assist you in making the decisions that are best for you.

When you are feeling sick or dealing with a diagnosis of any kind, making decisions about your health and life can be one of the hardest things to do. Which doctor should I pick? Which treatment should I do? Should I do chemo or not? Should I go the Western medical route or the natural route? Should I take that pill? Which diet is right for me? The questions just keep coming and everyone has different ideas of what you "should" do. It's so easy to get overwhelmed, confused, and terrified that you will make the "wrong" choice. I know this feeling well – it's paralyzing. This is where your heart and intuition come in big time and why it's key to get reacquainted. The answers to all these questions are within you. When you slow down, perhaps spend time in nature, cultivate practices that help you access your heart and elevated emotional states – like meditation and the HeartMath techniques such as the Quick Coherence Technique® in Chapter 6 – and connect with your Highest Self, you are better able to listen. Having a consistent daily morning spiritual practice is extremely helpful in beginning to reconnect with your heart and intuition (we will go over tips for an awesome morning practice in Chapter 12).

Here are four crucial things to remember when making decisions:
1 – Don't make any decision out of fear.
Decisions made from fear are never your highest and best choice. Return to a place of love, let the fear subside, and listen for the answer. So often we feel forced by doctors to make decisions and we do so in a terrified state. Don't be scared into a decision or afraid to take the time you need to make the best choice for you.

2 – Get still, trust, and follow through.

If you have a decision to make about your health, especially a big one, take some time to get still so that you can ask for guidance and listen more effectively. Don't forget to ask! This is really important especially if you are just getting reacquainted with your heart and intuition. Meditate and pray about it. Keep in mind that you may have to wait for the answer. It doesn't always come right away, but trust that it will and stay open to receiving it. And then when it does come, trust it and follow through.

3 – Your body talks.

One tool that my mentor taught me when making a decision was to listen to my body. She taught me to get really still, into a calm state by slowing my breathing, and ask the question I was seeking an answer to:

"Is it in my highest and best good to … ?"

And then I would feel into my body for clues. Feelings of openness, expansiveness, or tingling are clues that it is in alignment with my highest good. Feelings of constriction, tightness, or pain were clues that it may not be.

Or you may experience some sort of body sensation like a pain in the gut or headache that always happens when you have gotten off track. One of my clients describes a "twisting" feeling in her gut when she is about to do or is doing something that is not in her best interest or highest good. Listen to these body cues.

4 – Keep your mouth shut.

When you start talking to everyone you know about your huge dilemma you will inevitably get a lot of conflicting advice. It starts to get really confusing, really fast. Refrain from the urge to take a poll and get still, get calm, and go within first. Ask Source for guidance. You may be guided to talk to a certain person. Excellent. Go talk to that person, but avoid getting input from everyone you know.

Why should you trust your heart and intuition to guide you? This guidance comes from God – who is Infinite Power and synonymous with Love. The Creator of the cosmos also created you, loves you more than you can ever realize, and knows what's best for you infinitely more than you do or your parents or your best friend or any commercial or scientific study. It is by learning to get still, accessing the intelligence of the heart, and letting the fear fall away that we can hear our inner guidance, or what one of my favorite authors, Sue Monk Kidd, calls your "Big Wisdom," which I love. Answers don't always come as soon as you ask, nor are they heard with a booming audible voice or visible neon sign saying, "Go here, do that" (although that would be nice, wouldn't it?). Sometimes we must wait and have faith that it will come. It is in the waiting that so much growth and healing transpires. So, if you find yourself in this place of waiting, embrace it versus resisting it. The answer will come at the perfect time.

Source speaks to us in many ways – through those "gut feelings," a whisper in the stillness, words from a friend or stranger, a passage in a book, nature, signs, symbols, and synchronicities. One example of this is the purple tree story from Chapter 1. I sat in the park to pray and asked God to help me decide whether or not to do the mastectomy, even though in my mind I did not want to. However, the purple tree was a sign for me to move forward with the surgery and in my heart I knew that it felt right. The important thing is to keep your mind and heart clear and open to hearing the answers as they come. Meditation, stillness, and walks in nature can be very helpful for this. As you navigate your healing journey, drop into your heart, listen, and allow it to guide you. It knows the way.

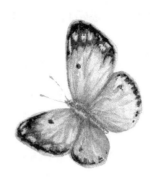

Chapter 12:

Where the Rubber Meets the Road: Practical Applications

"Knowing is not enough, we must apply.
Willing is not enough, we must do"
— Bruce Lee

Where the rubber meets the road is where concepts get put into practice and plans are set into motion. It may go without saying, but I'll say it anyway: you will only reap the benefits of what this book has to offer if you fully embrace this Whole-Hearted Healing approach and implement the 9 Essentials into your everyday life. Whole-heartedness is a mindset and way of healing and living that always takes into account the wholeness of who you are and focuses on living, listening, and leading with the heart.

Whole-hearted living requires action, contemplation, and discipline – not from a place of pressure or rigidity, but from a place of surrender, ease, intuition, trust, and the desire to heal and transform into the highest and best version of yourself. Sometimes the "doing" or the "action" is non-action or waiting for the next steps. Sometimes it's retreating within to ask your heart, waiting, and listening for the response. Keep in mind that "action" isn't always outward physical action. Sometimes action looks like being still, meditation, contemplation, imagination, prayer, or taking the time to feel your feelings and let them move through you.

In this chapter, I will highlight the important practices, tools, and concepts for you to apply on a *consistent* basis and ways to structure your life to support radical healing and transformation.

Make and Follow Your Self-Care Action Plan

In Chapter 10, we discussed the importance of self-care and encouraged you to create a Self-Care Action Plan. If you haven't already done so, take the time to create it and put it into action! Map out your daily, weekly, and monthly Self-Care Action Plan that outlines how you will best care for you – body, mind, heart, spirit – to support your healing journey.

As part of your daily routine, here are the basic things that I recommend including in some way: a morning practice (details discussed later in this chapter), some type of movement (Chapter 7), nourishing food (Chapter 8), hydration (Chapter 8), going to sleep by 10 p.m. (Chapter 7), getting sunshine/spending time in nature (Chapter 7), playing (Chapter 7), and doing something from your joy list (Chapter 10) every day. You may also include other things mentioned throughout the book and activities you enjoy or that you feel benefit your health.

As for your weekly and monthly self-care plans, create time for doing some of the deeper heartwork – looking at limiting beliefs and healing emotional wounds (Chapters 5 and 6). Maybe you realized you have several people to "Get Complete" with when we discussed the importance of this in Chapter 9. Schedule some time and space to do these things. You will only reap the benefits of these practices and exercises if you actually do them.

Create an Awesome Morning Practice

For anyone desiring to heal from chronic illness or transform their life in any way, a morning practice is crucial and one of the most important and effective things I recommend you commit to daily. Starting your day off with an awesome morning practice supports the health of body, mind, heart, and spirit – making it a super powerful tool that you definitely want to take advantage of. I recommend creating a practice consisting of the elements below, which will help you start getting that body hydrated, connect more fully to your heart and your emotions, allow you to become more aware of your thoughts, help you remember the Truth of who you are, and allow you to harness the power within to heal, cultivate more peace, and reduce daily stress.

There are five essential elements to creating an awesome morning practice that will help set you up for radical healing, peace, positivity and creating a life you love!
Start the day with:

1 – Hydration

As soon as you wake up, drink a large glass of water with lemon. This will help keep you hydrated, help flush toxins, and keep your bowels moving.

2 – Intention

Once you hydrate, look at yourself in the mirror and read your intention aloud three times. This is the intention you created in Chapter 4. Speak the words aloud with confidence and deep feeling as if it's already happened.

3 – Meditation/Prayer

Create a sacred space in your home for you to meditate/pray. It could be a corner of a room or even inside the closet. I had a client that had five kids and she created her sacred space in the closet. Make this your own private and special sanctuary. Place a comfy blanket or rug on the floor with a few colorful throw pillows, blankets, and a meditation cushion. If you can't sit on the floor, no problem, use a chair. Make this space one that you love to be in by adding crystals, a plant, sacred objects, a candle, or putting quotes or artwork on the wall. Do whatever you want to make this place special. It is here where you will go to meditate and pray. I also use my space to journal, reflect, or read.

I recommend that you start with five minutes of meditation daily and work up to twenty to thirty+ minutes and add in extra time for prayer. See Chapter 5 to see details on meditation.

Meditation and prayer is also the time to connect with Spirit. Take this time to remember who you are as a divine being, to feel the presence of God within and remind yourself of your innate ability to heal. It's important to consciously remind yourself of these things to ward off the fear and doubt that can so easily sneak in.

Here are a couple helpful affirmations you can say aloud or to yourself:
I am a magnificent expression of Divine Creation.
The loving Power that created me guides me and heals me.

4 – Activate Imagination/Vision

After meditation, take some time to look over your Whole-Hearted Vision Book that you created (refer to Chapter 4). Spend some time imagining yourself one year and five years from now as if you are already experiencing your vision and dreams fulfilled. Think and especially *feel* what it feels like to be vibrant and healthy (whatever that looks like for you) – perhaps it's having the energy to go kayaking or being pregnant with your first baby. Let those feelings wash over you. Remember, the elevated emotions + thoughts help you to connect with the Creative Consciousness to influence your reality.

5 – Gratitude

Write down five things you are grateful for in a journal. Include big and small things alike. Appreciation is a high vibration feeling that you will carry with you as you begin your day. See Chapter 6 for more about gratitude.

Other things you can include in your morning routine:
- A daily devotional reading
- Reading from a spiritual text
- Five to ten minutes of journal writing
- Essential oils – I love using essential oils as part of my daily routine for their full spectrum of physical, emotional, mental, and spiritual healing properties

Play around with these recommendations and customize a morning practice that feels like a good fit for you. The best morning practice is the one that you will actually do with consistency. You may find that you resist this idea. I've heard every excuse in the book. But, when my clients actually do this with consistency, the results are extraordinary and so vitally important to your healing, peace of mind, and happiness. And it's free, y'all!!

Six Superpowers

Throughout this book I've mentioned several practices or concepts that I like to call "superpowers" because when cultivated and practiced daily they are powerfully transformative, elevate your emotional state (which is key to healing), reduce stress, and invite more peace, connection, and happiness in your life. Make a point to activate these superpowers *daily*. Meditation/prayer, imagination, and gratitude are all part of my steps for an awesome morning practice, so if you do this you will have that covered. However, you can do any of these any time of the day.

1. **Meditation/prayer (Chapter 5)**
2. **Imagination (Chapter 4)**
3. **Gratitude (Chapter 6)**
4. **Heart coherence (Chapter 6)**
5. **Forgiveness (Chapters 6 and 9)**
6. **Surrender (Chapter 11)**

Concentric Living

Imagine concentric circles like the rings you see on a cross-section of a tree, a spider web, or a target sign. Concentric circles are circles that fit inside each other and share a common center. Smack in the middle is the epicenter and expanding out from there are layers of circles, also much like what you see when you throw a pebble in a pond and see the circles radiating outward. Symbolically, concentric circles represent wholeness and interrelationships. This is the perfect image to explain a powerful way to structure your life that cultivates healing and wholeness, as well as connection, inner peace, joy, and deep fulfillment.

The center of the circle represents your connection with God/Source and your own heart. This is the foundation of healing! Cultivating your connection with God and with yourself through your daily morning spiritual practice, doing your heartwork, and choosing to live, listen, love, and lead with your heart is the most important thing. When you do this, it will benefit all areas and relationships of your life like the pebble creating ripples in the pond. Creating space and time to show up every morning to do your morning practice, being in nature, doing the things that light you up and help you connect with your Higher Self and God will create a healing energy that affects you and your life in intangible ways.

This next circle represents your significant other. If you don't have one, no worries. But if you do, take time to cultivate love, connection, and good communication with your partner, which is key in your overall health and happiness.

As you move outward, the next ring represents an inner circle of women in your life that you can authentically connect with (in the truest definition of the word) on a soul-to-soul level. These are your chosen sisters. Cultivating sisterhood in your life is one of the most uplifting, transforming, supportive, and healing things you can do.

The next circle is your support team that we talked about in Chapter 9. This may include family members, a few close friends, practitioners, healers, coaches, and mentors that have agreed to support your healing journey, affirm your state of wholeness, and can hold the energy of love that is so important for healing. I highly recommend having a mentor or coach who can help you navigate your healing journey. It truly is one of the most supportive things you can do for yourself. Inevitably you will get scared, have doubt, move through challenging emotions, feel lost and overwhelmed, and have to make challenging decisions – a coach or mentor is super helpful to support you in this process.

Moving further outward to the next circle is your tribe. This is your community of like-minded friends (which can include family members) that you get together with for social gatherings, do fun things with, celebrate life with. These peeps are your clan that you can lean on for support when times get tough or you need a helping hand.

The most outer ring represents any community that you are a part of that is important to you, but may not be as intimate as the previous ones. These communities can be great for connecting with like-minded people in arenas that interest you, or that allow you to express your creativity and try new things. This could be a church community, book club, gardening club, gym, pottery class, dance class, etc.

Notice how I didn't include your family of origin here, because we are focusing on the relationships you choose. By structuring your life this way, your relationships with your family are likely to improve as you feel more grounded and connected to your Higher Self and with others.

Don't panic if you don't have all these concentric circles in your life right now. It takes time to cultivate and build these relationships. You first start with having an intention to create this. You must plant the seeds. Once the seeds are planted, you must water them and give them sunshine, which is the part where you take action, cultivate, and implement. Start with your own personal spiritual connection and morning practice first and then you can work on outer circles. It can take time, often requires action and almost always vulnerability to cultivate authentic connection, whether in partnership, sisterhood, or in finding your tribe. Be patient and hold the vision of feeling spiritually connected, fully supported, experiencing laughter, intimacy, joy, creativity, camaraderie, and authentic connection within your romantic partnership, inner circle of women, tribe, and community.

What does it feel like to "be seen, heard and valued, give and receive without judgment, and find strength and sustenance" from the relationships in your life?

What does it feel like to do life powerfully together with people you love and who love you?

What does it feel like to have people in your life that celebrate your victories, that remind you of your dreams and your Truth when you forget, and that are there at the drop of a hat to wipe the tears from your eyes?

Hold these visions and feelings in your heart and mind's eye. Be willing to take action to cultivate connection and stay open to new people and possibilities in your life.

Concentric living is about cultivating an incredible life of connection, love, belonging, and support and in doing so you are able to experience a deeper level of meaning, fulfillment, and richness in your life than you ever thought was possible. Consciously choosing to live in this way supports deep healing, more peace, fun, joy, creativity, adventure, courage, strength, confidence, and aliveness and is the blueprint for creating a life that you truly love!

Serve Others

Sometimes getting outside of yourself and your situation, no matter how dismal it may seem, and serving others can help dig you out of a self-loathing slump and can be profoundly healing. I believe one of the reasons we are here on this planet is to give our love and gifts to others. When we give our love away, we receive more of it, and it is this exchange that invites healing. Feeling sick and dealing with chronic illness can be very isolating if we let it and it's easy to get stuck in victimhood. It's easy to lose hope and perspective when we stay ruminating in our stories.

Back when I was sick and dealing with chronic rashes and fatigue I spent much of my time at home. I didn't want to go anywhere or do much of anything. I was beginning to feel like I was drowning and lost in a sea of my own negativity. I felt sad about my life, or lack thereof, and sad that I was not contributing to the world in anyway. I felt like I was suffocating and had to do something fast. One Saturday I passed a booth at the Farmer's Market looking for volunteers for an organization that provided housing for homeless people and taught them how to grow their food. Although hesitant, I signed up. The voice in my head tried to convince me the whole way home that it was a bad idea, that the people would stare at the rashes and that I wasn't "well enough" to do it.

I decided to do it anyway and volunteered once a month. It was such an amazing experience. It was just the medicine I needed to reconnect me with humanity and to realize I wasn't the only one struggling on this planet. I learned so much from the beautiful homeless men and women about resilience, heartache, struggle, and triumph. I didn't have to be perfect to love and help others. It was a powerful lesson. I gave my time and my love and received a hundred-fold return on investment – which is always how love works.

There's always a way that you can be of service in the world, in your family, in your job, and in your community (without depleting yourself). Find ways to share your love, your gifts, or even a smile. Being of service helps to open and heal your heart.

Be *You* and Love Yourself

One of the top five regrets people have as they move toward the end of their life is that they wished they had the courage to a live a life true to themselves and not what others expected of them.[70] The time is now to have the courage to live a life that is true to you and your heart. Like so many women, perhaps you've spent much of your life living to please others and doing what is "right" or "expected" from you. You've been programmed to push yourselves to the point of exhaustion and override your intuition and natural rhythms in order to achieve more, to be the good wife, good mom, good career woman, good lover, good friend, good daughter, good sister, etc. Did you lose yourself along the way? Perhaps you've gotten caught up in always doing for others, feeling the need to prove yourself – always striving, enduring, and trying to measure up. You've shoved your feelings under the rug and placed your dreams on hold for way too long. No more. Healing requires healing at the level of soul. Your soul is waiting for you to come home.

Remember that healing is about letting go of all that isn't Love and all that isn't the true you. There's no time to waste. It's time for you to reconnect with your authentic self, to love yourself as you are (scars and all), and get your power back. It's time to be you. Give yourself permission to let your soul shine, to feel deeply, to rest when your body tells you to, to scream when you are angry, to express yourself, to speak your truth, to feel all of your feelings, to make mistakes, to lead with your heart, to trust your intuition, to live full out, and to find your joy and share it with the world. Balance giving with receiving. Nurture yourself. Embrace your femininity and know that is your source of power and strength. Let go of putting so much pressure on yourself to be and do and allow yourself to feel joy and pleasure every day. Love and accept yourself for the extraordinary woman that you are. Be the imperfectly perfect you. If you don't know who that is, it's okay. I've said it before and I'll say it again: follow you heart, it knows the way.

Chapter 13:

What Gets in the Way

"Nothing is an obstacle unless you say it is."
– Wally Amos

It's inevitable that you will face some sort of obstacle or challenge when you embark on any meaningful and epic journey of healing and transformation. In my own experience of walking this Whole-Hearted path, as well as coaching others, there are some common things that keep women from being successful, detour them, or keep them from making the trek all together. I've included this chapter so you can be keenly aware of what may pop up so that you will be well-equipped and ready when it happens and courageously march on.

Just by reading this book you've already taken the first amazing step on your path to healing and wholeness. I've provided you with this Whole-Hearted Healing roadmap, but only you and you alone can make the journey. And the journey will be a powerful one if you choose to do it and do it whole-heartedly. Every essential in this book is just that – essential. These are essential pieces of the puzzle when it comes to health, healing, and living a life you love … one of more peace, love, joy, and connection.

Committing to addressing each one in your life can create powerful shifts and new possibilities for healing, growth, and transformation in ways that you may not realize until you've experienced them. It's important to delve into each essential with a spirit of curiosity, self-reflection, and openness and apply the tools, concepts, and strategies in each chapter with consistency and repetition to reap the benefits.

Now, let's talk about what gets in the way or may hold you back from fully experiencing the benefits of this Whole-Hearted Healing program.

Unwillingness to Change

I'm suggesting you make (perhaps for some) big changes in your life on many levels, and change can be uncomfortable. One thing I ask my potential clients before I agree to work with them is how teachable they are – how willing they are to learn and how willing they are to make changes in their life on a scale of zero to ten. I only work with people that are at an eight or higher. Why? Because these are the people that historically are willing to do the work necessary to make radical shifts and receive the benefits of healing and transformation my program is capable of. If you want your life to change, you have to be willing to change things in your life. It's that simple.

I had a client, Julie. She was a fifty-five-year-old nurse who complained of progressively worsening health, weight gain, digestive symptoms, acid reflux, fatigue, and high levels of anxiety. One of the most important things I do with my clients from the beginning is create a morning meditation practice, as well as teach techniques to help them begin the day in a coherent and calm state. As you've learned, chronic stress is linked to most every disease and therefore incorporating tools to manage your energy and inner state is paramount. Julie was reluctant and resistant to doing the five-minute meditation homework I gave her to do each morning before she went to work. When I asked her how her morning practice was going, she would tell me that she did it "sometimes," but said it was "hard" to do it every day and "hard" to get up earlier. And in the in next breath she complained about how "crazy" her life was, how she was always anxious, and admitted her digestive symptoms and acid reflux gets worse when she feels stressed. I was offering her tried and tested, science-backed tools to help her reduce anxiety and stress, but she was resistant and making excuses.

After three sessions of lack of compliance, we had a heart-to-heart. I asked her if she wanted to be free of the anxiety and digestive symptoms, etc. "Of course, I do," she told me. I re-explained the intimate connection between the physiology of the stress response in the human body and chronic disease. I also pointed out that by rolling out of bed and launching right smack dab into her perceived chaotic world that she was setting herself up for more of the same experience – anxiety and stress. I reminded her that she has to be willing to change things in her life in order for her life to change and for her desires and dreams to be made manifest! She finally began taking her morning practice and homework seriously and began to report decreased anxiety and improved energy levels within a short time frame.

We get so comfortable in our patterns of dysfunction that it's often difficult to change. You may find yourself being resistant to change as you move through these 9 Essentials. Just know it's normal to feel that way. But, bursting outside your comfort zone, being willing to change, leaning into that vulnerability of uncertainty, and trusting this process is where you begin to grow and heal. You can't keep doing the same things in your life (in your physical, emotional, mental, and spiritual world) and expect magically different results. It just doesn't work that way!

Here's a few mantras you can say aloud when you bump up against feeling resistant to change:
- I'm courageous. I trust, surrender, and flow with Life.
- I trust my heart to guide me. Peace of mind is mine.
- I open to fully receive all the good God has in store for me.

I Can't and It's Hard

The voice in the head or "ego mind" gets so loud at times that it's easy to get taken over by its messages. When you begin to make changes in your life you may bump into the seductive voice that likes to say, "I can't and it's too hard." I can almost guarantee this will come up several times on your journey. Just know it's par for the course. What's behind these persuasive thoughts? Fear. Fear that wants to keep you stuck inside the box that you live in and doesn't like things that are new or uncertain – it doesn't mind that inside this box you feel awful. You're afraid to fail, to change, to suffer, that you'll never get well or that you will get well, but it won't last. It's all too much, it's too hard and I can't do it, you tell yourself. And then you feel lousy, so to make yourself feel a little better you decide, "I'll do it when I feel a little better or have more time," which really means you're not going to do it, but you feel temporarily better about yourself for making a vague, some-day plan that deep-down you know you won't follow through with.

I admit, I've had my share of bawl-my-eyes out moments while feeling thoroughly convinced by the gremlin voices inside my head that I can't do this anymore and it's too hard! There were times when I felt this way going through a healing crisis while physically detoxifying my body, or as I was moving through a painful emotional wound from the past that needed to be released, or early on in my journey when I was craving sugar after I made the decision to ditch the cookies, cakes, and candy from my diet. There have been many moments of "I can't" and "It's too hard" over the years. Now I'm on alert for these spinster messages and I replace them with "I can and I will." I just switch them out.

When the "I can't" and "It's hard" messages pop up, it's helpful to remember a time that you accomplished something that you thought was too hard at first, but now can do with ease. For example, when I made the transition from getting off sugar and processed food and started eating grain-free, whole, real foods I had a couple of melt-downs. The first time I went to the store with my list in hand I walked in circles for two hours, was too overwhelmed, and left crying with no groceries. True story! Now, I've been eating this way for years and it's second nature. I rarely even need to pick up a recipe book anymore. I am able to make healthy food choices and recipes with ease.

I assure you that you absolutely can do this and it doesn't have to be as hard as you may think. I realized that so much of the stuff I immediately labeled as "hard," wasn't actually that hard and had to do more with my mind spinning out of control. Labeling something as hard over and over isn't helpful. However, it *is* helpful to think about the situation differently and make a choice to move through whatever challenge or goal with ease and picture yourself doing so. Take thing one at a time and consider the larger picture. For example, you may say getting rid of processed food and sugar is hard. If you keep this thought, "getting rid of processed food and sugar is hard," it will be. But, you know what's hard? How about dealing with all the pain, unpleasant symptoms, loss of function, worry, stress, or diagnosis that you may be facing right now? Doesn't living this way, with the possibility of things progressively worsening, seem harder than removing sugar and processed food?

It's important to know that healing, personal growth, and transformation are rarely linear. There will be dips and curve balls. I used to get all out of whack when a new symptom would pop up and often felt sadness that lasted for several days or weeks. I thought "oh no … this isn't working." But, that isn't necessarily the case. As we heal the toxicity (whether in mind, body, heart, or spirit) it has to come to the surface to be released and sometimes it's not a pleasant process. Don't lose heart. Healing emotional wounds and unearthing unconscious beliefs can be challenging. You may feel grief, despair, sadness, anger, rage, and a whole gamut of emotions you haven't allowed yourself to touch and feel. It's all perfect and necessary. Purge it. And remember to get the support and professional help you need to work through these things.

When you rub up against "I can't" and "It's hard," here's a few things to remember:

- Your Vision – Your vision for your health and your life is essentially your "why." Why go through things that are unpleasant or painful? Because you have a dream of feeling vibrant and healthy, of hiking the Grand Canyon, or of making a difference in the world. Remember, it's better to be pulled by your vision than pushed by your problems!
- Talk to someone on your support team or your coach who knows your vision and believes in your ability to heal. Sometimes you need someone to remind you why you are doing what you are doing, to remind you of the power you have within you to heal and offer love and encouragement.
- Take some time to have fun – do something on your joy list, watch a funny movie, dance, or just go have some fun with a girlfriend! And then circle back to the issue at hand. Sometimes taking a light-hearted break will help shift your thoughts and perspective.
- Choosing to be in a state of acceptance and surrender will bring more ease to the process.
- You can and you will. I believe in you. You've got this. Take it one thing, one moment, and one breath at a time.

Here's a few mantras you can say aloud when you bump up against "I can't" and "It's hard":

- I can and I will.
- I can do all things through God/Christ/Source who strengthens me.
- I choose to make this enjoyable and easy.

Quick Fix, Pill Popping Mentality

We have been conditioned – big time – to seek instant gratification and quick and easy fixes for what ails us. We have an entire medical system that offers pills for our ills – which may occasionally provide relief in the short term, but don't get to the root of the problem. While there may be a time and place for pills, we've come to rely on them for any and every unpleasant symptom we experience. We fail to take a holistic approach and seek our own intuition for guidance. If I would've had a little more awareness, I would've realized that those spicy hot wings I devoured in graduate school were doing a number on my digestive system and stopped eating them. What did I do instead? I popped an antacid and kept eating the spicy hot wings. A few years down the road I got incredibly sick, largely in part due to a leaky gut and poor digestion, which lead to a very weak and compromised immune system and a host of health challenges. Trust me, blindly popping pills for all your problems without addressing the whole person will not get you to thriving. I've personally experienced this and worked with patients in the medical system long enough to vouch for this one.

I regret to inform you that there isn't a "get healthy, lose weight, feel great, get happy, feel calm and centered, transform your life into epic awesomeness" pill. I wish there was. But, there's not. If your desire is to truly heal and create the life of your dreams, know that it will likely take some time, trust, commitment, and discipline. Discipline not in the "I gotta work so hard" sense, but setting aside time to cultivate and connect with your heart and implement nourishing practices. Having a pill-popping, "I expect results now" mentality, without doing much of anything, will totally block you from success with this program. The Whole-Hearted Healing process takes time and an investment in yourself.

The biggest complaint I hear is "I don't have time." Yes, you do. Sister, don't let that sneaky devil of a lie hold you back. You will always make time for what is important to you. And, you are oh so important … the most important! You cannot keep putting the needs of everyone and everything else in your life above your own. You being healthy and well allows you to serve other people, share your gifts with the world, and care for your family. Love yourself enough to do this. Being unwilling to take the time to *slow down* and delve into and integrate these essentials will hold you back from experiencing the extraordinary benefits from this program.

Yes, the 9 Essentials and many tools and suggestions in this book require time and discipline. You have to be willing to take the time to engage in your own self-care, create a morning practice, feel your feelings, question your beliefs, cultivate connection, seek out quality food, create a vision, move your body, and incorporate the many other important recommendations in this book. All I can say is that it's so worth it! Instead of moving through these essentials like to-do's that have to be checked off a list, engage your heart and *enjoy* the journey. Through this process I was able to discover my true authentic self for the very first time and begin truly living and loving from my whole heart. It changed my life. I think deep down we all desire that. Don't let quick-fix conditioning and lack of immediate results hold you back from beginning or continuing your Whole-Hearted Healing journey.

Here's a few mantras you can say aloud when you feel frustrated by not getting results quickly enough:
- I trust in my body. I listen to my body. I allow my body to heal.
- Slow down. Breathe. Relax into this moment.
- I choose to enjoy the journey.

Skimming Over Simplicity

There are many simple tools and strategies in this book that you may have heard thrown around before in the self-help/healing world – things like self-care, self-love, feel your feelings, create a vision, ditch sugar, or get plenty of sleep. I find that sometimes clients skim over the simple stuff because they think it's too simple to fix their "big" health problems and don't *actually* do it. Dialing in all these foundational things add up to significant shifts and healing.

You may be tempted to blow off one or some of the essentials and recommendations and deem them as unimportant because they are simple or maybe you already kinda did that once. Sure, I get it. The 9 Essentials provide a holistic approach to healing and thriving, so each one is important and works synergistically with the others.

As always, I recommend listening to your intuition and heart when it comes to making changes for your health, but at the very least spend some time with each essential and give it a shot before you discard it. Every essential has its importance and has been just that – an essential piece for many women restoring their health and creating deeper and more meaningful lives. Not everything has to be overly complex and cost a zillion dollars to be effective. Consistent meditation can reduce or eliminate anxiety, depression, and pain often similarly or more effectively than prescription medications without the awful side effects. Sunshine, nature, eating real food, laughing, dancing, and taking the time to connect authentically with yourself and with the people in your life has healing benefits in ways that can't be measured. You may have the tendency to want to skim over the simple stuff or give a half-hearted effort. Go all in with your *whole* heart when it comes to each essential and embrace the simplicity. I love this quote:

> *"It is always the simple that produces the marvelous."*
> – Amelia Barr

Here's a few mantras you can say aloud when you are trying to make things too complicated:
- Keep it simple, sexy.
- I delight in the simple things of life.
- Mastering the basics is key.

Don't Let Anything Hold You Back!

Awareness
One of the best ways you can be sure to avoid these obstacles and keep them from getting in your way or holding you back is *awareness*. Now

that you are aware of what the common obstacles are, you will be more likely to spot these stealthy sabotaging scoundrels if they arise and be able to say "thanks but no thanks … I'm moving forward and I'm committed to my vision of health and all the things I'm choosing to have and experience in my life."

Remember Your Vision

Don't forget to use your vision to pull you out of your overwhelm, doubts, discomforts, "I can't," "it's hard," "I don't have enough time," "it's scary to feel my feelings" … all those thoughts that hold you back from all that you truly deserve and desire. Pull out that vision book, drop into your heart, and feel that feeling of your wish fulfilled. Oftentimes remembering your dream or "why" you are doing something is the very thing that keeps you moving forward!

Take It One Essential at a Time

Another hack that will help ensure your success is to take things one essential at a time. When people start trying to take on multiple essentials at one time they get overwhelmed and don't fully integrate each particular topic into their lives. At the same time, please understand that you will continue to go deeper and deeper into some of these essentials over time. Essential #4: Feel Your Feelings, for example, discusses the importance of healing your emotional wounds when it comes to chronic health issues. Will you heal all emotional wounds in one journaling session or one EFT tapping session? No. You've gotta peel back those layers, and over time you will continue to heal deeper layers and have more insight, awareness, and understanding as you continue to commit to your healing process. But for now, you will begin to build your awareness of your feeling world, learn some of the tools to help you process them, and improve your emotional intelligence. Spend a week or two on each essential and then move on to the next. You can circle back to any one of these essentials as you feel called to go deeper.

Accountability = Success

Lastly, the other hands-down, best way to avoid detours and get the best results is accountability. If you can find someone to help keep you accountable as you move through the 9 Essentials (or even read this book and implement them with you) it can not only help you avoid these obstacles but help ensure your success. We are much more likely to do something and be successful at it when we have support and are accountable to someone. When we tell another human we are going to do something and we know that person is going to check in and ask us if we did it, we are much more likely to do it! Many of my clients say that it's so much easier implementing things like a morning practice, uncovering subconscious beliefs, and making nutrition and lifestyle changes when I am holding them accountable, giving them feedback, and when they are able to talk through things and ask questions.

You Can Do This!

Now you know the top things that get in the way of you experiencing more health, healing, vitality and success with this program. Use these tools, mantras, and your awareness to keep these potential obstacles from getting in the way of all that you desire. You can do this! You've got the map, now all you need to do is put one foot in front of the other and begin the journey!

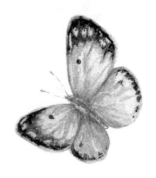

Chapter 14:

Conclusion

"A woman is the full circle.
Within her is the power to create, nurture, and transform."
— Diane Mariechild

Embracing a whole-hearted life involves living and loving from your whole heart, listening to it, and allowing it to lead. This is a journey focused on true healing or returning to wholeness and relating to yourself as a spiritual, mental, emotional, and physical being. Whole-hearted living is a never-ending path of self-discovery in which you come more fully into remembering and reclaiming yourself as a magnificent expression of divine creation. The infinite power of God that orbits the planets around the sun, turns a caterpillar into a butterfly, and created the intricacies, uniqueness, and vibrant colors of the plant and animal kingdom is also inside you — never forget this. Identifying with this Truth of who you are aligns you with your innate power within to heal.

Navigating through these 9 Essentials unlocks a path to healing and wholeness that doesn't end when you finish this book, but only just begins. However, now you have a roadmap that leads you into deeper levels of health, wholeness, peace, joy, connection, and love. I found each essential to be a key element in my journey (and so many others) of healing and transformation of body, mind, heart, and spirit. Take the time to delve into each one with a spirit of openness, curiosity, and navigating with your intuitive heart.

Essential #1: Taking Responsibility for Your Health

This essential discussed the importance of taking responsibility for your own health and life. You are currently dealing with a health challenge – how will you choose to respond? When you are able to accept what is happening in your life, an opening for possibility and receiving something new and different surfaces. Could this disease presenting in your currently reality be the catalyst for radical growth, transformation, and creating a life that you love? It can be if you choose it. That's what this program is all about.

Essential #2: Creating a Vision: Harness Your Power to Heal

This essential helped you learn how to create a vision and intention for your health and how important this is in harnessing your power to heal. Hopefully by now you are beginning to realize that you are constantly creating your life through your beliefs, thoughts, words, and feelings. By consciously creating a powerful intention and vision for your health and life *and* thinking, feeling, and aligning yourself with this vision *daily* you begin to tap into your ability to co-create your reality in the direction of your heart's desires.

Essential #3: Thoughts and Beliefs

This essential dove further into the power of your thoughts and beliefs and how they shape your everyday experience. Perhaps you realized that you were still operating by core beliefs that were formed in childhood that you may no longer agree with and are in direct contradiction to what you truly desire! These limiting beliefs, like software programs running on a computer, have been powerfully influencing your life in negative ways, but the good news is that once you become aware of them, you can change them. You've also learned that the thoughts you think impact your reality. When you attach and identify with negative and repetitive thoughts, you begin to call those experiences into your life, whether you realize it or not. Healing and transformation require challenging your core beliefs and becoming aware of the thoughts you think and aligning them with Truth, Love, and that which you desire to most experience in this life.

Essential #4: Feel Your Feelings

This essential created awareness around the importance of your emotional health and the extraordinary power your feelings have in your ability to create your life experience. Feelings are energy that are meant to be fluid and fully felt. Addressing emotional wounds by moving through stored, stuck, and stagnant low vibration emotions such as resentment, fear, and grief must be addressed in order to fully heal and thrive. This is often one of the biggest blocking factors when it comes to health. Cultivating emotional intelligence on a daily basis, giving yourself full permission to feel your feelings, and having tools to process and move your emotions is key to being well.

Essential #5: Live to Thrive: Key Lifestyle Factors

This essential dove into incredibly important lifestyle factors for you to incorporate on a daily basis that are crucial for healing and thriving. Getting enough quality sleep in the prime-time window is important for healing. Making time each day for a movement/exercise routine, getting safe sun exposure, and letting nature nurture you are simple yet powerful healing strategies. Taking time in your life to play and laugh helps to reduce stress, elevate your emotional state, and cultivate healing. A happy heart creates a happy body! Reducing the number of toxins you are exposed to on a daily basis by making changes in your home environment and personal care product usage is critically important to decrease stress on your body while healing and for long-term well-being.

Essential #6: Eat, Drink, Detox

This essential discussed the importance of thinking and relating to the food you eat as "medicine" and focusing on whole, quality, nutrient-dense foods while avoiding toxic and inflammatory ones. Remember, it's not all about what you eat, but how well you can digest, absorb, and assimilate the food you eat. Digestion is key to a healthy body and immune system, therefore incorporating strategies to optimize your digestion is important. Hydration and detoxification are also important ways to keep your body healthy and must be addressed daily.

Essential #7: Connection and Relationships

This essential discusses the importance of cultivating authentic connection in your life and how to do it, as well as the power of sisterhood, the importance of having a support team and getting complete in your relationships. Everyone wants to feel seen, heard, and valued and having relationships and opportunities in your life where you can connect authentically is powerfully healing, uplifting, and creates a life of deeper meaning and fulfillment. Getting complete with the people in your life by telling them how much you love or care for them, apologizing for past hurts you may have caused, or forgiving people and letting go of holding on to stored up resentments, guilt, hatred, and anger invites healing for you, your family, and anyone involved. Relationships can be the source of deep emotional pain and turmoil. Focusing on healing the relationships in your life or letting go of certain ones may be crucial to your healing.

Essential #8: Love Yourself

This essential is one of the most important essentials of them all. It's all about loving yourself and how to start doing it. These symptoms you are experiencing in your body are often a reflection of what is happening on the inside. Whatever challenging situation you find yourself in right now, use it as an invitation to fall back in love with you, to remember your True Nature and to reconnect with your heart. You are a holy and divine daughter of God – already whole and complete as you are. You knew that when you were born, you just forgot. We all did. The time is now for you to remember and reclaim this, to truly love yourself again, and to care and nourish yourself. No one can do this but you. Your self-love is your medicine for yourself and for the world. What does it really mean, look, and feel like to truly love yourself? Dive into this question and explore it fully. Don't skim over this one!

Essential #9: Trust and Surrender

This essential ties everything together by reminding you that at the end of the day healing and wholeness requires that you must trust and surrender. Trusting your heart, the God-within, and surrendering to Love to guide and heal you is the path to peace and is a daily choice and practice. It's so easy to forget that we can let go and choose to surrender the pain, the hardship, the fear, the overwhelm, the doubt, the suffering, the anguish, the grief, and the confusion because we are so used to carrying it for so long. Breathe and let go, my love. If you can begin to trust and surrender your life, your decisions, your future and each and every moment to the Divine, you will inevitably experience more freedom, peace, clarity, and wholeness.

My Wish for You

From my heart to yours, it is my deepest desire that you will choose to use this experience that you find yourself in at this very moment in time – no matter the severity of symptoms, disease, health challenge, or label you've been given – and begin to see this as a portal of transformation and opportunity to bring you back to your heart, to love yourself again, and to experience wholeness. When you focus your energy and effort on desperately trying to get rid of the symptoms or fighting the disease, you often further perpetuate that which you desire to be free from and miss the underlying message, gift, invitation, and opportunity it brings to invite radical healing (for body, mind, heart, and soul) and transformation.

Remember, true healing and "conquering chronic illness" really is about a return to wholeness – being "well in your soul." It's not about fighting against disease, or just about getting rid of symptoms (although that can and often happens) or avoiding death, because none of us will. Death is not the end, it's a continuation. Each of us have a finite time on this planet. Some of us will live to our nineties or one hundreds and some of us will be called to transition well before that.

My wish for you is that for the remainder of time that you have on this planet that you will know what it means to be whole, to love yourself exactly as you are, to love your life, to be the full authentic expression of you, to love fiercely and live full out, to give your gifts to the world, to grow, to experience life to its fullest, and to live whole-heartedly. My wish for you is for you to experience health in your body, peace in your mind, love in your heart, and joy in your spirit.

This Whole-Hearted Healing journey requires a certain degree of action, contemplation, soul-searching, heart work, and perhaps for you to show up differently in your life. Before you do anything, make the commitment to begin to listen, love, and lead with your heart versus your head. It takes practice. And begin to shift your thinking and approach to health and life by acknowledging that you aren't just a physical body, but that you are complex and dynamic and have an emotional, mental, and spiritual body as well. Remember, you are a spiritual being having a human experience. Next, review the obstacles and where the rubber meets the road section so you can be aware of what common road blocks pop up along this journey and what things are important to implement on a day-to-day basis. Now, begin to implement each of the 9 Essentials with commitment, discipline, openness, curiosity, compassion and ease and enjoy the journey.

You've probably realized that each of the 9 Essentials are big topics that go deeper than I could fit in one book, which is why I created my Whole-Hearted Healing coaching program to guide women through this process. I absolutely love being witness to a woman's healing journey, the alchemical process of transformation – from caterpillar to butterfly. I believe that supporting and coaching women through their healing and transformation process is part of the reason why I'm on this planet and why I have walked the path I've walked. The journey isn't always easy – every woman's journey is unique to them, and support is often crucial for success.

I've provided you with the healing roadmap and many tools for your journey. You are equipped to make headway on your own. However, I personally have found having a mentor and coach to be essential, exponentially easier, and more impactful than navigating this often complicated and challenging journey of life on my own. Being able to talk with, and process through things with someone who had been where I was before and who had journeyed through their own health challenges was priceless. Having someone to point out my blind spots, to see things I could never see on my own, and having someone to keep me accountable was and is key for me to stay focused and make epic strides in my health and life. Regardless of how you choose to proceed on your healing path, trust and listen to your heart … always.

And don't forget that you are magnificent, my love, truly extraordinary, and always guided and provided for. All the love, healing, and answers you've been seeking are already inside you, because Divine Love resides within. Love yourself. Trust in your body's ability to heal. Trust your heart. Listen. And follow through.

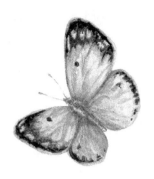

Acknowledgments

I never had any particular desire to write a book. I remember a few years ago I went to see an extraordinary and very intuitive healer named Deva. After the session, she told me one day I would write a book and speak in front of a lot people. I looked at her like she was nuts and dismissed it entirely. And then cancer happened and I made the commitment to listen and live from my heart versus my head. My heart led me many places. It led me back to myself and it led me to writing this book.

Over the past couple years, I began to get nudges to write a book and a calling to be a stand for women desiring to heal and thrive. I tried to dismiss it at first, but the nudges kept coming. "Okay God," I said, "I don't know anything about writing a book. So, if you want me to do this you are going to have to show me how." I knew it was time to quit my job to birth something new, perhaps a book, but I wasn't sure. I quit my job in February of 2018 and within weeks Dr. Angela Lauria and the Author Incubator showed up in my world. Months later this book was birthed. Thank you, Angela, for helping me get my story and message to all the beautiful women of the world! I couldn't have written this book without you and your team!

I have tears in my eyes in this moment as I write this thinking of all the angels, teachers, and healers that graced my presence and supported Chad and I during my healing journey. I couldn't have walked the courageous path I've walked, nor written this book, without the support of many.

To the Morgan James Publishing team: Special thanks to David Hancock, CEO & Founder for believing in me and my message. To my Author Relations Manager, Bonnie Rauch, thanks for making the process seamless and easy. Many more thanks to everyone else, but especially Jim Howard, Bethany Marshall, and Nickcole Watkins.

Thank you to Dennis and Kristen Notten, Ron Banuelos, Dr. Matthew Buckley, Deva Ruebenheimer, Fran Bell, Dr. Chris Holder, Dr. Joseph, Michelle Longo O'Donnell, Melissa Raymond, Dr. Véronique Desaulniers, Arttemis Keszainn, Susan Naziri, Lana Boyuk, Dr. Basa, Dr. Kim, Reverends Brian and Kristen Grandon, Reverends Steve and Mary Bolen and my entire team of doctors, healers, counselors, and teachers that supported the healing of my body, mind, heart, and spirit.

To our Tribe, our dear friends and chosen family –thank you for your love and support through thick and thin and everything in between. Thank you for crying with us, celebrating life with us, and being extraordinary lights in the world.

Women of Radiance – you are my soul sisters in every sense of the word. Thank you, Trina, Cora, Lindsey, Deanne, Mallory and Kristen, for being the wind beneath my wings, always lifting me up and always being there no matter what. And to all my dear, dear sisters – especially Amanda, Andi, Amy, Kelly, Amber, Ruth, and Denise – thank you for loving and supporting me throughout this journey. To all my sisters (including those not mentioned) – you are each a source of strength, healing, and inspiration to me. I love you all! I'm deeply grateful and honored to walk through this life with each of you.

Thank you, mom and dad for always being there, loving me, and supporting my decisions, no matter how unconventional. Mom, thank you for staying with us and helping me recover from surgery. Thank you,

Marlene and Chuck, for loving and supporting me like I am your own daughter and for providing a place for us to stay when we didn't have one. Thank you, Brian, Bobbi, and Chris for your love. Thank you to my nephews Hunter, Spencer, and Harrison for making my heart happy when I see your faces. Maya, my fur baby girl, thank you for always being a steady stream of joy and light in my life.

Thank you to my husband, Chad – my strong, wise tree. God couldn't have fashioned a more extraordinary partner for me to do this life with. Thank you for being so stinkin' strong during the storms of life and always seeing and affirming my wholeness. Thank you for reminding me who I am when I forget. Thank you for loving me fiercely, making giant leaps of faith with me, encouraging me to write this book and always believing in me. I love you infinitely.

Lastly, I thank God for bringing me back home to mySelf and my heart. Thank you for my healing and this opportunity to share my story and learnings. And thank you for the knowing that You are within me, always guiding me, and that I'm always loved and provided for. I love you.

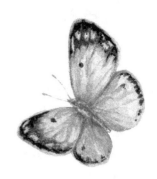

About the Author

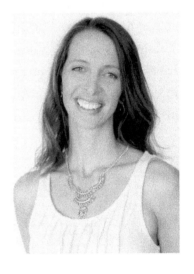

D r. Brenda Walding is a Holistic Wellness & Transformation Coach and specializes in supporting and empowering women to truly heal and thrive. Brenda spent the past decade dealing with chronic health challenges, including life-threatening infections, chronic rashes, and breast cancer. After having to go on disability due to rapidly declining health in her late twenties and not getting results or relief with Western medicine, Brenda began exploring natural and holistic medicine. Through changes in diet and lifestyle and incorporating natural healing remedies and modalities, she began to gradually restore her health. She became laser-focused and committed to studying holistic healing in order to further regain her vitality.

Years later, her experience of breast cancer was the catalyst for her to heal not only on the level of body, but mind, heart, and spirit as well.

Cancer called her to dive deep, reconnect with her heart, and to finally begin fully living and creating a life of her dreams. Brenda is passionate and committed to helping other women to do the same.

Dr. Walding is a women's holistic health advocate, Doctor of Physical Therapy, and holds several certifications in the realm of natural and holistic healing. These certifications include: Functional Diagnostic Nutrition practitioner, TaoFlow yoga teacher, and HeartMath Certified Coach. She also co-founded NativePath, a popular nutrition and lifestyle company.

Brenda currently resides outside of Austin, Texas on the beautiful Lake Travis. She loves spending time in nature, connecting with her husband, family (including her beloved mini Goldendoodle), and friends, cultivating community, sitting in sacred circles with women, and learning about holistic healing and spirituality.

Websites: www.brendawalding.com, www.sickofbeingsickbook.com

Email: risetoradiance@gmail.com

Facebook: https://www.facebook.com/drbrendawalding/

Instagram Handle: http://instagram.com/brenda.walding

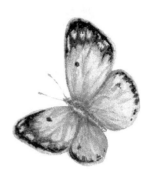

Thank You, Beautiful!

Thank you so much for reading this book and being committed to your own healing path! I truly believe that when one woman heals herself, she plays an integral role in the healing of all the women on the planet!

FREE VIDEO MASTER CLASS: As a token of my appreciation and for additional support on your journey, I've created a video master class that highlights and reviews the Whole-Hearted Healing approach and the 9 Essentials.

Go to www.sickofbeingsickbook.com/master-class to access it.

Sending you love and healing hugs,

Brenda

"Every woman who heals herself helps heal the women who came before her, and all those who come after her."
– Dr. Christiane Northrup

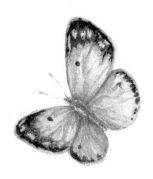

References

1   https://www.ncbi.nlm.nih.gov/pmc/articles/PMC2515569/

2   https://chriskresser.com/the-dangers-of-proton-pump-inhibitors

3   McCraty, Rollin, Science of the Heart, Exploring the Role of the Heart in Human Performance Volume 2. HeartMath® Institute. 2015. www.heartmath.org.
And
McCraty, Rollin, The Energetic Heart: Bioelectromagnetic Interactions Within and Between People. HeartMath® Institute. 2003. www.heartmath.org.

4   Dispenza, Joe. Breaking the Habit of Being Yourself: How to Lose Your Mind and Create a New One. Carlsbad: Hay House, 2012.

5   Miller, Lyle, Alma Dell Smith. The Stress Solution: An Active Plan to Manage the Stress in Your Life. New York: Pocket Books, 1993.

6   Dispenza, Joe. Breaking the Habit of Being Yourself: How to Lose Your Mind and Create a New One. Carlsbad: Hay House, 2012.

7   McCraty, R., Atkinson, M, & Tomasino, D. Modulation of DNA Conformation by Heart-Focused Intention. HeartMath® Institute. 2003. http://www.aipro.info/drive/File/224.pdf

8   http://www.masaru-emoto.net/english/water-crystal.html

9   Braden, Gregg. The Spontaneous Healing of Belief: Shattering the Paradigm of False Limits. Carlsbad: Hay House, 2008.

10   https://www.healyourlife.com/how-i-healed-myself-after-breaking-6-vertebrae

11   Braden, Gregg. The Spontaneous Healing of Belief: Shattering the Paradigm of False Limits. Carlsbad: Hay House, 2008.

12   https://www.ncbi.nlm.nih.gov/pmc/articles/PMC2515569/

13   http://www.superconsciousness.com/topics/science/interview-dr-bruce-lipton

14   https://www.equilibriume3.com/images/PDF/The%20Research%20of%20Candace%20Pert.pdf

15   https://www.ncbi.nlm.nih.gov/pmc/articles/PMC4398234/https://www.sciencedaily.com/releases/2012/04/120402162546.htm

16   Grossarth-Maticek, R. and H.J. Eysenck, Self-regulation and mortality from cancer, coronary heart disease and other causes: A prospective study. Personality and Individual Differences, 1995. 19(6):p.781-795.

17   HeartMath® Institute. 2012. The Math of HeartMath / Coherence. https://www.heartmath.org/articles-of-the-heart/the-math-of-heart-math/coherence/

18   McCraty, Rollin, Science of the Heart, Exploring the Role of the Heart in Human Performance Volume 2. HeartMath® Institute. 2015. www.heartmath.org.
     And
     Childre, D., Martin, H., Rozman, D., & McCraty, R. Heart Intelligence, Connecting with the Intuitive Guidance of the Heart. HeartMath. 2016.

19   https://www.equilibrium-e3.com/images/PDF/The%20Research%20of%20Candace%20Pert.pdf

20   Wiley, T.S, Brent Formby Ph.D. Lights Out: Sleep, Sugar and Survival. New York: Pocket Books, 2000.

21 https://www.ncbi.nlm.nih.gov/books/NBK19961/

22 https://www.ncbi.nlm.nih.gov/pubmed/26300312

23 https://www.ncbi.nlm.nih.gov/pmc/articles/PMC1402378/

24 https://bjsm.bmj.com/content/43/2/81.short

25 http://articles.mercola.com/sites/articles/archive/2016/06/29/
    vitamin-d-insulin-resistance.aspx
    https://www.ncbi.nlm.nih.gov/pmc/articles/PMC2290997/

26 https://articles.mercola.com/sites/articles/archive/2016/06/29/
    vitamin-d-insulin-resistance.aspx
    https://www.ncbi.nlm.nih.gov/pmc/articles/PMC5440113

27 Ober, Clinton, Stephen Sinatra, MD, Martin Zucker. Earthing:
    The Most Important Health Discovery Ever! Laguna Beach: Basic
    Health Publications, 2014.

28 Li, Q. 2009. Effect of forest bathing trips on human immune func-
    tion. Environmental Health and Preventive Medicine. 15(1): 9–17.
    https://link.springer.com/article/10.1007/s10086-008-0984-2

29 https://www.ncbi.nlm.nih.gov/pubmed/24682001
    https://www.omicsonline.org/open-access/effects-of-laughter-
    therapy-on-anxiety-stress-depression-and-quality-of-life-in-cancer-
    patients-1948-5956-1000362.php?aid=60533
    https://www.cancercenter.com/treatments/laughter-therapy/

30 https://www.medicalnewstoday.com/releases/9681.php

31 Fitzgerald, Randall. The Hundred-Year Lie: How Food and Medi-
    cine Are Destroying Your Health. New York: Penguin Group, 2006.

32 Fitzgerald, Randall. The Hundred-Year Lie: How Food and Medi-
    cine Are Destroying Your Health. New York: Penguin Group, 2006.

33 https://www.ncbi.nlm.nih.gov/pmc/articles/PMC4798150/

34 https://www.medicalnewstoday.com/articles/221205.php

35 Desaulniers, Véronique. Heal Breast Cancer Naturally: 7 Essential
    Steps to Beating Breast Cancer. TCK Publishing, 2014.

36 U.S. Environmental Protection Agency. 1987. The total exposure assessment methodology (TEAM) study: Summary and analysis. EPA/600/6-87/002a. Washington, DC.

37 https://www.huffingtonpost.com/entry/synthetic-chemicals-skin-care_us_56d8ad09e4b0000de403d995

38 Fitzgerald, Randall. The Hundred-Year Lie: How Food and Medicine Are Destroying Your Health. New York: Penguin Group, 2006

39 https://www.nrdc.org/stories/dirt-antibacterial-soaps?gclid=_EAIaIQobChMIs-jh8JOY3QIVFndeCh2dtAMZEAAYASAAEgJk_hfD_BwE

40 http://www.iarc.fr/en/media-centre/pr/2011/pdfs/pr208_E.pdf

41 http://www.bioinitiative.org/ https://www.ncbi.nlm.nih.gov/pubmed/26300312

42 https://www.ncbi.nlm.nih.gov/pubmed/12479649

43 https://nutritionj.biomedcentral.com/track/pdf/10.1186/1475-2891-3-19.

44 Morse, Robert. The Detox Miracle Sourcebook: Raw Foods and Herbs for Complete Cellular Regeneration. Arizona: One World Press, 2012.

45 https://www.ewg.org/foodnews/strawberries.php

46 https://www.ncbi.nlm.nih.gov/pubmed/17916947

47 https://www.seafoodwatch.org/consumers/seafood-and-your-health

48 https://www.usatoday.com/story/news/nation/2014/02/03/added-sugars-heart-disease-death/5183799/

49 https://www.dhhs.nh.gov/dphs/nhp/documents/sugar.pdf

50 https://bmjopen.bmj.com/content/6/3/e009892.full.

51 Wolf, Robb. Wired to Eat: Turn Off Cravings, Rewire Your Appetite for Weight Loss, and Determine the Foods That Work for You. New York: Harmony Books, 2017.

52 https://www.marketplace.org/2013/03/12/life/big-book/processed-foods-make-70-percent-us-diet

53 https://universityhealthnews.com/daily/heart-health/oxidized-cholesterol-vegetable-oils-identified-as-the-main-cause-of-heart-disease/

54 https://www.ncbi.nlm.nih.gov/pmc/articles/PMC4524299/

55 http://drhyman.com/blog/2010/06/24/dairy-6-reasons-you-should-avoid-it-at-all-costs-2/

56 Morse, Robert. The Detox Miracle Sourcebook: Raw Foods and Herbs for Complete Cellular Regeneration. Arizona: One World Press, 2012.

57 Cordain, PhD, Loren. The Paleo Diet: Lose Weight and Get Healthy by Eating the Foods You Were Designed to Eat. Hoboken: John Wiley and Sons, Inc., 2012.

58 https://www.ncbi.nlm.nih.gov/pmc/articles/PMC3471010/

59 https://www.ncbi.nlm.nih.gov/pubmed/23850261
https://articles.mercola.com/sites/articles/archive/2017/08/29/aspartame-health-risks.aspx

60 https://www.nrdc.org/issues/toxic-chemicals

61 http://www.organic-systems.org/journal/92/JOS_Volume-9_Number-2_Nov_2014-Swanson-et-al.pdf

62 http://www.nongmoproject.org/learn-more/what-is-gmo/

63 https://www.ncbi.nlm.nih.gov/pmc/articles/PMC2515351/

64 https://www.ewg.org/tapwater/state-of-american-drinking-water.php#.W1jSvBJKjOQ

65 https://www.ncbi.nlm.nih.gov/pubmed/26156538

66 https://hippocratesinst.org/wheatgrass-juice-benefits

67 https://www.ncbi.nlm.nih.gov/pubmed/14518774

68 https://draxe.com/matcha-green-tea-burns-fat-and-kills-cancer/

69 Holt-Lunstad, J., Smith, T. B., Baker, M., Harris, T., and Stephenson, D. (2015). Loneliness and social isolation as risk factors for mortality: A meta-analytic review. Perspectives on Psychological Science, 10, 227-237. https://scholarsarchive.byu.edu/cgi/viewcontent.cgi?article=3024&context=facpub

70 Ware, Bronnie. The Top Five Regrets of the Dying: A Life Transformed by the Dearly Departing. Balboa Press, 2012.

Printed in the USA
CPSIA information can be obtained
at www.ICGtesting.com
JSHW022212140824
68134JS00018B/1018